THE NO MORE
EXCUSES DIET

THE NO MORE EXCUSES DIET

3 Days to Bust Any Excuse,
3 Weeks to Easy New Eating Habits,
3 Months to Total Transformation

MARIA KANG

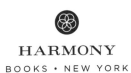

HARMONY

BOOKS • NEW YORK

Copyright © 2015 by Maria Kang

Published in the United States by Harmony Books, an imprint of the Crown Publishing Group, a division of Random House LLC, a Penguin Random House Company, New York.
www.crownpublishing.com

Harmony Books is a registered trademark, and the Circle colophon is a trademark of Random House LLC.

Library of Congress Cataloging-in-Publication Data is available upon request.

ISBN 978-0-553-41967-2
eBook ISBN 978-0-553-41968-9

Printed in the United States of America

Book design by Rae Ann Spitzenberger
Interior photographs by Mike Byerly
Jacket design by Jess Morphew
Jacket photograph by James Patrick

10 9 8 7 6 5 4 3 2 1

First Edition

TO MY MOTHER, CAROLINE KANG,
FOR BEING MY BEST FRIEND
AND INSPIRATION

CONTENTS

INTRODUCTION

What's YOUR EXCUSE for not having the body that you want? Are you unmotivated, tired, or frustrated? Do you lack time, energy, finances, or support? What's holding you back? What's preventing you from being healthy, fit, and confident?

There are so many different ways to answer those questions. If you've been on this roller-coaster ride before, then you know what I'm talking about. You love food. You're too tired. You lack energy. You have no willpower. You don't have time—and the list goes on. I know exactly how you feel.

But these are *excuses.*

Excuses validate our choices. They let us off the hook and give us permission to fail. While psychologically soothing, excuses limit our ability to create opportunities to progress toward personal health. What if I told you that the only thing standing in the way of you and the body you want is a single excuse? Would you confront it? Would you commit to overcoming it? That's what this book is about. I want you to bust through these excuses and empower yourself. I want you to rewrite your story and feel empowered to be anybody you want to be. Are your excuses valid? Sure, some of them probably are. Can most excuses be overcome? Absolutely.

This book is not about making you feel guilty for how you look, or ashamed of the choices you've made. This book is about getting you to a place where you love your life, love your body, and love your health. And in order to feel that way, you have to bust through the excuses that might stand between you and your best body. That's what we will do together over the course of this program.

We will review your excuses, combat them, then attack them. I provide a simple set of rules to follow that will have a revolutionary impact on your ability to achieve your goals. I also present simple and flexible ways for you to understand fitness, nutrition, goal setting, and time management. Not only do I give you some simple workouts and easy recipes that make fitness feasible, but I also offer a maintenance plan for your new normal—the person you become when you've taken the path to fitness and good health. After all, it is often harder to stay in shape than it is to get into shape.

As a busy working mom of three young sons, who were born in 2009, 2010, and 2011, it wasn't easy for me to get back into shape. After giving birth to my first son, I gained 35 pounds, my muscles were gone, and my midsection looked like a deflated balloon. Regaining my physical fitness was hard. In fact, it was really hard. There were days when I needed to wake up at the crack of dawn to fit a workout into my schedule. There were days when I was tired or unmotivated, when the last thing I wanted to do was prepare the day's lunches and dinners so my family and I would have healthy foods at hand. But even when I had no energy or I felt overwhelmed by my responsibilities, I pushed myself to do it anyway. Sure, there were times when I missed workouts, slept in, or splurged on a piece of chocolate cake. But I never gave up. I never lost sight of my goal: getting into the healthiest shape I could.

Reaching any lofty goal isn't going to be easy—and if you think this No More Excuses plan is going to be a cakewalk, then let me tell you right now that it will not be. But setting a goal for your health and achieving it is *worth the effort*. Whether your aim is to fit into a certain size pants, to eliminate a health risk, or to change your energy level, reaching that goal will make you feel physically, mentally, and spiritually *amazing*.

The first step in realizing your fullest potential is to make a *choice*. We make a thousand choices every day that either help or hinder us in becoming successful in reaching any weight-loss goals. After all, we know eating fried and sugary foods is unhealthy, we know physical activity is vital, and we know we can really make fitness fit into our lives if we truly want it there. Busting your excuses boils down to figuring out what you really want. Why is this endeavor important to you?

It's important because this is your own path and your own body. This vehicle isn't going anywhere until you get into the driver's seat. Once you know your *why* for wanting to attain your best body, figuring out how to do it becomes easy. You need to identify the reasons that will keep you disciplined in this journey, and then make it your choice to prioritize your goal, no matter what obstacles arise.

And obstacles will arise. All of a sudden, it's pizza night at home. It's a lunch potluck at work. You feel lack of personal support. You catch a cold or burn the midnight oil working. Your life gets busy, your efforts become half-hearted, and your results—well, there's not much in the way of results. I have been on this path more times than I can count, but I'm here to tell you that *you can break away from that path*.

I want to help you develop your own No More Excuses plan to take your life to the next level. This book isn't (just) about how to eat right and exercise. It is also about learning how to achieve the goals you've set for yourself, no matter what else is going on in your life. It's about believing in your abilities and giving yourself permission to succeed. It's about getting to know YOU: your strengths, your weaknesses, your excuses, and, most of all, your motivation.

Motivation is the *key principle* in this journey. If you examine the lives of those who are in incredibly good shape, you will see an invisible energy constantly pushing them to stay disciplined and train harder. That energy is motivation. They might be motivated because their career depends on their physical body and beauty, as is the case with so many celebrities and models. Or maybe they're motivated because their personal identity is tied to having a fit body (the way athletes need to be incredibly fit to succeed). For us "normal" people, though, motivation comes from setting higher expectations for ourselves and in believing we can meet those expectations.

Over the course of this program, we are going to examine what motivates you, and we are going to clear away the distractions that get in your way.

Some of you might want to look amazing in an outfit, or be able to walk confidently into a room without feeling physically insecure. Others might want to get healthier to avoid diseases or escape the torment you felt as a child for being overweight. No matter what motivates you, the first step in achieving your goal is to take action and identify your motivations, whatever they may be, and create a way to hold yourself accountable. This is not about shame or guilt; nobody is going to scold you if you don't succeed. This is about understanding your motivation, embracing your goals, and realigning your world to succeed.

Let me tell you about some of the things that have motivated me. In my early twenties, I feared childbirth would destroy my body. I was a young and athletic personal trainer who won several beauty and fitness contests. At the gym, older women would constantly react to my fit physique by saying, "Wait until you have children...."

So after I gave birth, I was motivated to prove that motherhood didn't have to change me and I could even make myself better. I created a flexible but disciplined workout and diet plan, executed with persistence and reflected on weekly—and it worked!

Another motivation was my desire to feel confident in my skin. In my mid-twenties I struggled with binge eating and I watched my weight balloon. My metabolism was damaged from years of yo-yo dieting, and my weight no longer responded to any diet or exercise program. It was exhausting to run, my clothes didn't fit, and I was embarrassed to go swimming. I wanted to feel sexy, firm, and fit again. I was motivated to achieve the firm body I'd had in my early twenties and avoid the frustration I felt in being overweight by my mid-twenties. I was motivated by the pleasure of success and the pain of failure.

You need to be, too.

Imagine how confident you will feel, how healthy you will look, and how happy you will be when you create for yourself the body and health of your dreams. You set out with a goal in mind and you achieved it. I *know* you can do this. Why? Because I've done it and I will show you how to do it, too.

There are three cycles to this program. They are cycles because you can repeat them or move from one to the next as you're ready:

1. **The S.P.E.E.D. cycle**
2. **The S.T.R.I.V.E. cycle**
3. **The S.C.O.R.E. cycle**

The S.P.E.E.D. cycle is your liftoff. Within the first three days of the program, you will create a game plan complete with goals, a timeline, a reward, and a map. This is when your motivation is high; you will develop a fitness and diet program specific to your body, your lifestyle, and the goals you want to achieve. With S.P.E.E.D., you are setting the goals, planning the journey, envisioning the outcome, executing the plan, and delivering the results on a weekly basis. The goal is to get to the finish line quickly and efficiently.

The S.T.R.I.V.E. cycle is your operative phase. This is the period where you will not only be creating new habits for a healthier life, no matter what, but you'll also be following a diet and exercise schedule that you've tailored to your specific goal. S.T.R.I.V.E. is not just about stepping up your lifestyle to attain a goal; it's also about developing the technique to stick with the plan no matter what. Once the initial motivation dissipates, attaining goals becomes more difficult. This is natural to the process, so do not be discouraged by it. Instead, S.T.R.I.V.E. will teach you to push through it!

During this cycle you will be mastering your ability to look challenges in the eye and not give up. You will overcome addictive foods and come face-to-face with the excuses that are preventing you from following through to achieve your dream. I provide strategies to help you bust down those excuses so that you can rise to greater heights than you thought you could achieve. With S.T.R.I.V.E., you are seeking the issue, tackling the problem, reflecting on failure, identifying the cause, visualizing a new route, and engaging in a new action. Your goal is to keep pushing until you reach your objective.

The S.C.O.R.E. cycle is your success phase. You've maintained your three-day momentum, then spent three weeks developing healthy habits, and now you've reached the three-month mark—and have officially hit your target. This isn't the end, though; this is the beginning of other goals to reach that lie just over the horizon.

Many people lose weight only to regain the weight slowly afterward. That won't happen to you with the No More Excuses program because this third cycle combats complacency and adjusts your life to a new normal. With S.C.O.R.E., you reflect on what made you successful and celebrate your journey. This is also when your program is in operational mode and you are rejuvenating after the hard work you've put in these past three months. When you achieve your goal, it's a time to reflect, rest, and evaluate where you go from here. What's your new goal going to be now? It's to make fitness an official lifestyle so you can proudly improve your best body, every year of your life.

I will help you understand how your body works and aid you in developing a fitness routine that blends strength, cardio, and flexibility training, so that you get the most out of each minute. These easy at-home workouts include different levels of fitness, depending on your experience and your energy level, so that you have options, no matter what else is going on in your life.

I also provide a balanced meal plan based on a 30 percent carbohydrates, 30 percent protein, 30 percent fats, and 10 percent flexibility philosophy that will help you make sure every meal you eat is well balanced and fills your body with the ingredients it needs to function and stay energized. This plan encourages you to consume balanced meals throughout your day. I haven't eliminated major food groups, and I even leave room for a couple weekly treat meals.

Oftentimes, we allow our family, our job, or our responsibilities to overwhelm and distract us from caring for ourselves. This No More Excuses program will bring you back to yourself. You will uncover your internal warrior in this weight-loss battle. You will learn how to balance your life, prioritize your health, and feel whole again.

Can you imagine how amazing your body will look and feel in just three months?

Getting fit requires desire, discipline, and dedication. If you are ready to forfeit your excuses and take the plunge, this book is for you. You will achieve your fitness goals if you make a personal promise to not give up until you get there. This mentality makes success a matter of "when" you will reach your goals and not "if" you will reach them.

I'm not going to coddle you. This plan isn't easy. It takes effort. It will take time, too, but I guarantee you: You will become healthy if you make the choice right now to never give up. No More Excuses!

PART 1

WHAT IT'S ALL ABOUT

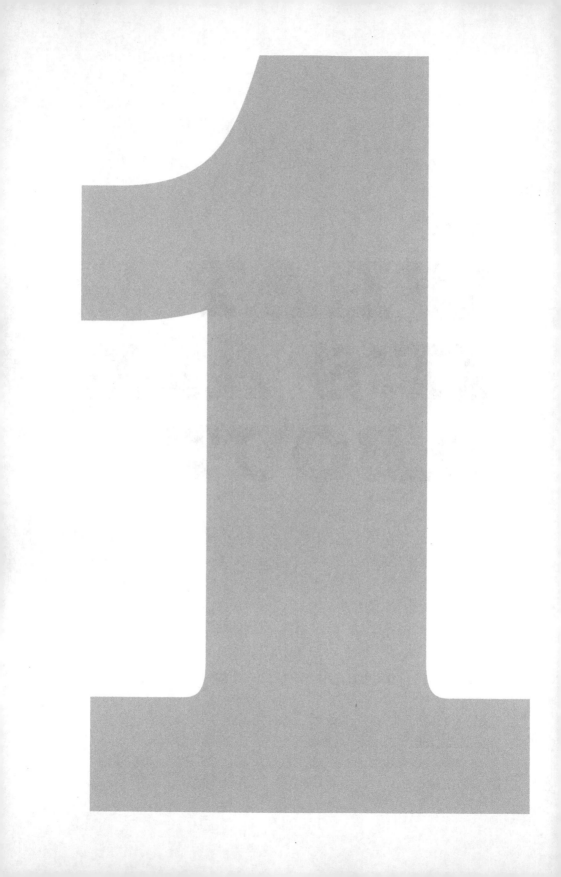

MY STORY

I wasn't always fit. I never played a sport, and I grew up eating sugary cereals, boxed dinners, and fast food. I don't have superior genes, either. As the eldest of three daughters, my heavier frame always mimicked the bone structure of my overweight mother. While my mother was a charismatic, vibrant, and successful businesswoman, she didn't apply that same drive to maintaining a healthy lifestyle. She became a diabetic in her twenties, experienced strokes in her thirties, and had heart attacks and a kidney transplant in her forties.

Watching her suffer made me vigilant about protecting my health. At twelve years old, I purchased a cheap Reebok workout video by Gin Miller at my local store, and I used old phone books as my fitness stepper. I read the many diet books that my mother had around and began following a diet comprising foods with no fat, such as candy, breads, and pasta. After slowly gaining weight in my teens, I began to experiment with other diets. I attempted a juice fast—that lasted only one day. I attempted the Atkins diet, but after three weeks of beef patties, bacon, and no bowel movement, I quit that, too. I tried diet pills and weight-loss shakes, with no success, either.

In college, I ecstatically became a part-time personal trainer and finally began learning how the body worked. I discovered strength training, integrated it into my workout routine, and was seeing incredible results. I learned how to master my metabolism by performing strength and cardio exercises, consuming balanced meals every three hours, and enjoying a splurge meal once a week. While it was difficult training, working, and studying all at the same time, I made it work because I was so conscious of the health risks that were inherent in my family. I was able to graduate in four years with a double major in history and international relations and a minor in political science from the University of California at Davis.

During my transition to work life, I decided to challenge my body and I started competing in local beauty and fitness competitions. For weeks, I would follow a strict diet of lean protein and complex carbohydrates, coupled with intense strength training and cardio exercise. I wasn't eating enough calories for my activity level, though, and after each contest I would binge eat; I biologically and psychologically needed to refuel. I did win several contests locally and nationally, but I felt a void.

I was in my early twenties. I had graduated from college, moved to San Francisco, broken up with a long-term boyfriend, and changed occupations. I had built an award-winning physique and was even featured in national magazines. I should have felt happy, satisfied, and accomplished—but I didn't. I felt empty.

I felt like I didn't know who I was and what motivated me to be independent, ambitious, competitive, and fit. In those reflective moments I could hear my mother's voice, cheering me on, supporting my efforts and celebrating the things I was able to do because she couldn't.

Filling the Void

Up to this point, I thought that attaining objects, titles, and money would make me happy. But it didn't. In fact, nothing did. I felt empty, so I began filling that emptiness with things that had consoled me in the past. I started consuming cakes, cookies, chocolate, ice cream, and candy. While I ate upward of 3,000 calories per sitting, it seemed my body didn't register my incredible intake because I never felt physically satiated. When guilt overtook my psyche, I forced myself to throw up. I would begin this destructive cycle of bingeing and purging up to three times a day, three or four times a week for several years. Dominated by thoughts of inadequacy, feeling spiritually vacant, and lacking control of thoughts, I found that people and events around me created intense anxiety. My weight crept back up to my early college days, and my self-esteem was declining quickly.

I remember going home one day and admitting my eating disorder to my mother. She confessed that she understood my personal plight intimately, as she also suffered from bulimia when she was younger. In a *Twilight Zone* moment, I felt that history was repeating itself—after all, eating disorders leave a genetic stamp.

I saw the first twenty years of my life pass me by, and in an instant I grasped how every choice I had made was influenced by my mother's pushing me to become everything she couldn't be (because she had married young, had multiple children, and was overweight). I realized that I didn't have ownership of my decision to pursue extreme fitness and live independently and successfully in a big city.

My obsession to compete and win at all costs had been motivated by a desire to make my mother proud. She sacrificed her youth and her health in both raising us and working. She didn't take time for herself; she couldn't pursue a more fulfilling life because her health limited her. One night, I started writing a letter to my mother—the woman for whom, beginning in fifth grade, I used to wake up each morning at 5 AM so I could iron her clothes, cook her breakfast, and pack her a healthy lunch. Even then, I knew her busy life prevented her from making the healthiest choices, and I had grown up wanting to help her live a healthier life. I felt a piece of me shatter every time I saw her inject insulin, take prescription medications, or become briefly paralyzed from a minor stroke.

I didn't want to become my mother, but whether I knew it or not, I already had.

Finding My Passion

My crazy eating led me to gain 30 pounds in one year. My clothes no longer fit, and the extra pounds weighed heavily on my nearly 5-foot-4-inch frame. I started living in comfortable yoga pants, large skirts, and empire-waist dresses. I knew my body was metabolically damaged from years of disordered eating. It didn't know when I would feed it, or if the food I consumed would remain there. I felt like my body was literally grabbing every calorie and saving it for a future famine.

In the depth of my personal pain I started to write, read, reflect, and pray. I began a personal website to document my innermost thoughts and initiated connections with people who empathized with my story of fear, guilt, shame, happiness, and triumph. I realized that I needed to let go of the past, to stop thinking of the future, and to start living in the present. If I consumed a cookie, I let it digest without negatively thinking of becoming fat or my feeling ashamed for lacking self-control. If I had an out-of-control binge session, I didn't beat myself up about it, and instead I determined to make more careful choices. I let go of my shame, reflected on what had caused the action, and held myself accountable for the consequences.

During this time I discovered similar stories of women who had been on yo-yo diets, taken weight-loss pills, and tried fasting, only to be left with bodies that didn't trust their owners anymore. Our bodies didn't feel loved, nurtured, or protected. We were treating our bodies like the enemy.

So I began the process of loving my body again. I nourished it with healthy, whole foods. I strengthened it through physical movement. I cared for it by giving it enough water, sleep, and rest. I reminded myself daily that however my body manifested through good nutrition and exercise, it was beautiful. So it manifested at 145 pounds—20 pounds over my goal weight—for many years. In one of those years, 2007, I met my future husband and I created my fitness nonprofit, Fitness Without Borders.

After years of battling the bulge, I had realized being healthy was important to me. I knew it could prevent health-related diseases like heart disease and diabetes, as well as improve the quality of my life. I saw these changes in other people, in the low-income places I worked, in the elderly people I served, and in the overweight groups I mentored. Fitness was a powerful, life-giving force that I genuinely had a passion for, yet like everyone else I still struggled daily with my personal excuses.

Whenever I was bored, anxious, or stressed, I binged on chocolate and chips. If I was depressed, I often skipped workouts and opted to lie in bed. Even when I began eating well and exercising consistently, my body was unresponsive. I told myself that my mother's genetics had finally caught up with me, that there was nothing I could do to lose those 20-plus pounds to get back into the shape that I loved. I resisted going on any diet because I knew it would trigger an eating disorder.

A part of me was settling down at my new weight, and I began believing this was as good as it would get. But part of me also knew that it was just an excuse. Deep within, I knew I could build my best body again if only I was willing to put in the effort.

In 2008, I found out I was pregnant, and I spiraled down into a state of depression for the majority of the pregnancy. Though my partner and I were engaged, we were unmarried. I had just quit my corporate job in San Francisco and moved home to Sacramento to help care for my mother, who was undergoing dialysis treatments for kidney failure. Not only was I fearful of our future together, but I was uncertain of what pregnancy would do to my body—a body still struggling to lose those 20 pounds. Most mothers in my family had experienced weight gain, stretch marks, excess skin, swollen ankles, enlarged feet, and deflated breasts—and many of those conditions didn't go away after the babies were born. I was not too excited about my own pregnancy, therefore.

I wanted to maintain some feelings of control, so I began journaling my food intake and ensuring that I consumed only 500 additional calories per day. I maintained a light workout routine and I gained weight slowly. In those moments, I could almost feel my relationship with my body changing. Whereas before I had felt disconnected or at war with my physical form, now I was seeing it in a new light. I began revering my body for being the vessel containing this little miracle growing inside me. Wow, I could grow a human life!

By the end of my first pregnancy, in January 2009, I was 180 pounds and gave birth to a healthy 7-pound, 14-ounce baby boy. After his birth, I continued my healthy lifestyle by dropping my caloric intake slowly and adjusting my workout routine to match my son's sleeping and nursing schedule. Within six months I was down to 10 pounds below my pre-pregnancy weight! I was shocked to be in the 130s again, but not as shocked as I was when I discovered I was pregnant with baby number two.

This time, I wasn't as anxious; I knew that it was possible for me to have a healthy baby and take care of myself at the same time. I began my pregnancy routine of managing my schedule, eating whole foods, splurging on occasion, and exercising one to three times a week. By the end of my second pregnancy in April 2010, I had gained 37 pounds and delivered in a record-breaking time of one hour after admission to the hospital.

My days were now busy with nursing my youngest son, attending to my eldest, and working as a business owner of small residential care facilities for the elderly. I knew I wanted to add one more child to our fast-growing family. By this time, David and I were married. We settled into my hometown of Elk Grove, California, and I was becoming a local leader as the founder of my fitness nonprofit Fitness Without Borders; I also was leading a free "mom fitness" group. We welcomed our third son in December 2011.

Life was incredibly busy; I was multitasking as a business owner, nonprofit director, freelance writer, and mother of three very young boys. Despite my daily obligations, I made it a priority to incorporate a workout routine that gave me energy and made me feel great. I was careful to take in enough food to keep my metabolism churning through the day. My weight loss was slow, but each week I was getting a little bit closer to my goal of feeling confident in a midriff-baring workout outfit.

Reaching a daily sweat was important for me because it was the only "me time" I had anymore. I looked forward to my workout session, whether it lasted 20 minutes or an entire hour! Exercising raised my self-esteem, increased my stamina, and lifted my spirits. I made a plan and set a deadline of six months to get back into great shape. I was doing something for myself, an action my mother inadvertently taught me to appreciate.

My long-term goal was to have a toned midsection, feel confident in a tank top, and weigh in at 125 pounds again—a number I hadn't seen for ten years. I raised the stakes by booking a profes-sional photo shoot. To keep me motivated and stay the course, I created short-term, achievable goals that allowed me to feel suc-cessful. Six months after my doctor gave me clearance to exercise, I was brimming with pride. I set a goal, I followed a plan, I overcame adversities, and I followed through. I showed my husband a woman he'd never seen before, and I proved to friends that it was possible to improve your body after having a child.

Above all, I was a good role model for my children. They saw me prioritize my health without sacrificing my work or family life, and they observed how energized and happy the exercise and good eating habits made me. Not only was I able to complete my fitness goals with a balanced approach, but I also got the body I wanted in a smart, healthy, and sustainable way.

What's Your Excuse?

As I got ready to post my new photos to my website and Facebook page, I thought about what I wanted to say. I was proud of how I looked, and I was even more proud of all the work and commitment that had brought me to that point. I had vanquished a lot of per-sonal demons to get to the healthy, happy relationship I now had with fitness and food. I once believed that it wasn't possible for me to have a body I loved. I had thought that there was no way to avoid the health issues that plagued my mother. I had let fear stand between me and the healthy lifestyle I wanted. After my pregnan-cies, though, I had stopped letting all of those excuses get in my way. I had committed myself, one day at a time, to reach my goal, and one day at a time I had achieved that goal.

In posting those photos, I wanted to share my revelation: that the only thing standing in the way of success is an excuse, a rationalization for why we sometimes can't follow through. I titled my newest image of myself with a popular fitness catchphrase, "What's Your Excuse?"

I've always struggled with weight, both before and after motherhood, and I know how tough it can be to achieve the body you want to have. My caption was meant to be taken literally: *What is your excuse?* What is holding *you* back from being the best and most healthy person *you* can be? I wanted to inspire others, to make people realize that it's possible to overcome the obstacles that stand between them and their goals.

That single caption, posted on a photo of me and my three kids, captured 16 million views within two weeks on Facebook. The image was featured on dozens of morning shows, evening shows, talk shows, and news shows. I was interviewed on *Good Morning America, Today,* and CNN, as well as on programs in Australia, Germany, the Philippines, Ireland, and Canada. I was mentioned in *Time* magazine's People of the Year issue. In three weeks, my Facebook page attracted more than 260,000 new members and my website traffic ballooned to more than a million views.

I was shocked.

My question stirred a controversy, and my character as a mother, wife, and fitness enthusiast was put on the line. Some people accused me of being a bad mother for supposedly working out all day. Others complained that I had great genes, a full-time nanny, or a rich husband. People thought my image was faked or that my children were paid models because it seemed impossible that I could get these results without sacrificing motherhood, time, and resources. Yet despite some of the backlash, thousands more were inspired. I received emails from people who had decided, for the first time in years, to start prioritizing their health. Even though many responses came from single parents, working two jobs or recovering from past injuries, they were tired of excuses holding them back from having the bodies they wanted. My question was their wake-up call.

These viewers saw that if I can do it, they can do it, too. Thousands of women joined the online community, and in less than four months, hundreds of "No Excuse Moms" groups popped up in more than twenty-nine countries. People began celebrating non-scale victories, like fitting into their favorite jeans, wearing a bikini at the beach, and completing a 5K run. For many, it was the first time in their lives they had set a goal, created a plan, and achieved that goal.

And so can you.

Many people think being healthy is as simple as calories in, calories out. But it's more involved than that. In between today and the day you achieve your goal is a long road that's littered with a lot of excuses. You need to be prepared. You need to know what to do when you get confused, sore, tired, busy, stressed, depressed, unmotivated, and overchallenged. You need a simple how-to fitness and nutrition guide that won't leave you with "analysis paralysis" every time you step onto the gym floor.

I'm here to teach you what I have learned to do mentally and physically to get into great shape. The first lesson is the *power of choice*. After all, your ability to create a thought and proceed with an action will determine your results. Whatever choice you make, whether it's to run three miles or to splurge on a chocolate chip cookie, you just own it. You decide if it helps or hinders your long-term goal, then you create an action plan when that challenge arises again.

Every action begins with a choice.

Whether you're facing a public struggle or a private one, I show you that it's possible to achieve your goals, that you can have the body you want and the health you deserve, no matter what obstacles are in your way.

Your body is the only personal vehicle you will own in this life. So honor it. Respect it. And let it amaze you with everything that it can do when you give it the care it deserves!

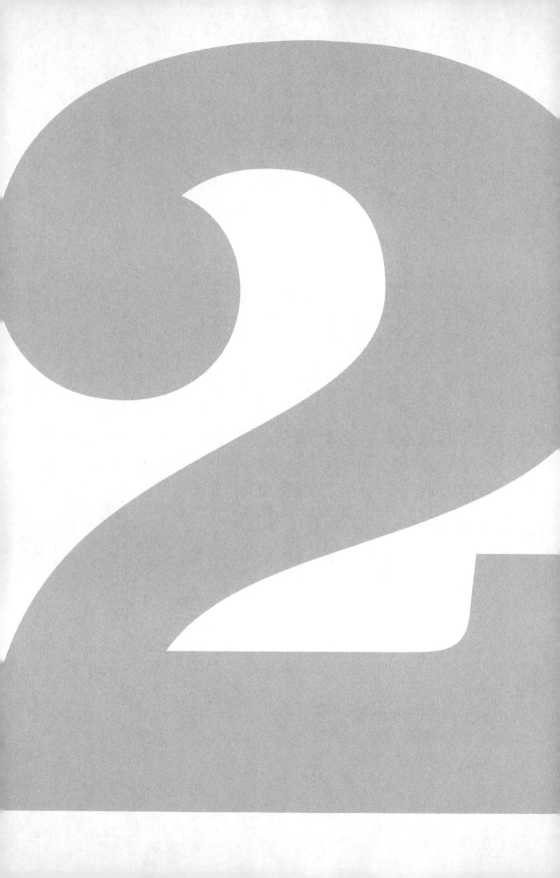

THE POWER
OF THREE

One of the top excuses that people have for giving up on a diet or health goal is that they aren't getting results. And while I've designed this program for you to start basking in success quickly, you need to know that it's going to take time and effort to get the final results that you want. And that's okay—that's how it's supposed to work! It takes three days to overcome a craving and bust your excuse, three weeks to develop a new good habit, and three months to see a physical transformation. Reaching these milestones in your fitness journey will give you patience and perspective as you endure the process of changing your actions to produce a new, best body.

The Three-Day Rule

Think back to all the times you tried to diet and exercise in the past. What held you back from becoming your best self? Did you get busy? Did you give into cravings too many times? Was it too unrealistic a goal? What was your excuse?

Let's examine some of the excuses that have been holding us all back from living a more fulfilled life. (In Chapter 9, I talk more about excuses and give you strategies for busting through them.) Here's a sampling of the biggest problems I have heard from the thousands of women I've helped.

PAST EXCUSE #1: *"I have no time to exercise."*
SOLUTION: *Commit to a set time.*

I like a long night's rest as much as anybody, but nothing feels like "winning" more than getting up early to work out, clean up, and prepare for work, all before 9 AM. There are a lot of benefits to being an early riser. Not only do you get your priorities out of the way, but the house is quiet, the streets are empty, and often the sun hasn't risen yet. It's empowering to spend a few silent minutes in this serene environment and envision the day you have planned. If mornings are truly not going to work for you, commit to training during your lunch break or immediately after work. Wherever your opportunity to train fits in your day, commit to it for three days. By the fourth day, I promise it will start to feel like second nature.

PAST EXCUSE #2: *"I love eating."*
SOLUTION: *Eat fewer refined carbohydrates.*

Like many people, I grew up eating sugary cereals, white rice, fruit roll-ups, and boxed dinners. Saying that I love carbohydrates is an understatement. I used to eat rice with spaghetti or macaroni and cheese, and I even added some rice to my ramen noodles. When I started learning about macronutrients in college, I realized my diet needed a major overhaul, and I committed to stop eating rice. The first few days were hard, especially because anything that was savory needed—according to my taste buds—some rice for balance.

But after three days, the rice craving was not as great. After a couple weeks, my taste buds regenerated and I didn't want rice much anymore.

PAST EXCUSE # 3: *"I hate exercise."*
SOLUTION: *Master your weakness, enjoy your strengths.*

I'm not a big runner; running brings me back to my childhood embarrassment at running a mile on a dirt track in middle school and vomiting my SweeTARTS soon after. Gross, I know. Every time I run, my body feels heavy and my heart feels overworked. I know, however, that in order to step up my fitness game, I have to incorporate running. So, whenever I need to get back on track, I start by running 2 miles at a moderate pace. I don't worry about how fast I'm going, and I don't panic when my body feels weak and breathless. If it's too difficult, I focus on taking a short water break every 5 minutes or I walk uphill instead of run. As long as my heart is challenged for 20 minutes, it doesn't matter if I'm sprinting, jogging, or walking fast—my body is working hard and I don't quit; that's all that matters. The next day, I do it again. By the third day, my body is starting to adjust to this new activity and I can begin extending my distance or increasing my pace.

Completing a difficult cardio challenge applies to every type of cardio exercise, not just running. If you find swimming, stair-climbing, spinning, or jumping rope especially difficult, then focus on that weakness. When you do what your body feels is challenging, you become stronger because your mind and body are both engaged in the activity.

PAST EXCUSE #4: *"I'm afraid of failing."*
SOLUTION: *Visualize success.*

The three-day rule can have a huge impact on people who have been pessimistic about past weight-loss journeys. It allows you to adequately prepare by reading this book, creating a support network, and acquiring accountability tools. In the first three days, you reflect on your excuses, affirm your strengths, and create action plans to combat those excuses. One of the main messages in this book is the power that comes from envisioning your success and focusing on what you desire. So take this opportunity to let go of what scares you and instead focus on what inspires you.

PAST EXCUSE #5: *"I have no discipline."*
SOLUTION: *Find a healthier alternative.*

There was a point in my life when I had several friends who loved to meet over coffee, which meant drinking a lot of fancy coffee drinks. It became such a habit that even when we weren't meeting, I found myself making a trip to the café for my fix. Eventually, I found myself consuming 400 extra calories a day and spending $25 a week on coffee. When I realized this was becoming an addiction, I made a conscious effort to thwart this consumption. At first I ordered unsweetened tea, then I took just water. After just three days, I started becoming mentally stronger to make healthier drink choices. Not only was my waistline decreasing but so was my spending!

If you are addicted to a specific food—like sweets, breads, or cheeses—abstain from it for three days and you'll find that the craving will dissipate. I'm a big chocolate lover. There was a time when I felt a meal wasn't complete until I ordered dessert! It wasn't uncommon for me to order dessert before the main meal, just to ensure I saved room in my tummy for it. When I realized my love for chocolate was impeding my physical results, I grew conscious of this craving and resolved to deal with it. Even though my body and mind wanted my routine dessert after dinner, I didn't give in for three days. By the fourth day, my body was feeling lighter and my mind felt stronger.

So remember this: If you have trouble performing any routine, do it without fail for three consecutive days, and by the fourth day it will become easier. You can use this three-day rule to reshape nearly all your habits and routines.

PAST EXCUSE #6: *"I lose my motivation."*
SOLUTION: *Create a meaningful goal.*

To give meaning to your efforts, you need to find value in each action. If you are unmotivated to work out or to eat healthy, perhaps you haven't landed on the deep, desirable reasons this journey is important to you. Do you want to avoid health-related issues like heart disease, diabetes, and stroke? Do you want to grow old with your children or feel sexy around your spouse? Figure out why this effort is important for you, and have those reasons on hand every time you lose motivation. If you need to, take a mental break; but by the third day, start taking action. If you wait any longer than three days, complacency moves in and takes hold.

Do any of these excuses sound familiar? Believe me, I know how real they sound; you are not alone if one—or a few, or all—of these excuses applies to your life. But I make you this promise: *These are not permanent obstacles.* You *can* overcome them, without giving up those family, friends, and responsibilities that are so important to you. It's all about change—change in your perspective; and in my experience, that change takes three days to become established.

Just focus on making a change in the next three days, and a new habit will kick in. The first day you are living more consciously will be difficult, and so will the following day. But, by the third day, and especially by the fourth, the change will seem natural. We are creatures designed to adapt, and the first step in adaptation is changing an action that sends you in a purposeful direction. Just don't set too many goals at one time. Master one change, then move on to another.

I've used the three-day rule in several parts of my life, from breaking my addiction to rice, to carrying a water bottle everywhere I go. I focus on getting through the first three days, and after I have overcome the initial challenge, the action becomes habitual.

The Three-Week Rule

If you consistently practice a new routine for twenty-one full days, you will establish a whole new lifestyle. Healthy habits are the building blocks for your success. They are the difference between having to actively choose to do a routine and simply living it.

FIRST PHYSICAL TRANSFORMATION

Besides marking your habit-forming ease, the three-week mark is also the first time you will measure yourself after your initial weigh-in. I make it a general rule to not expect significant physical results before three weeks. Once that twenty-first day arrives, though, that's when you break out the measuring tape and step on the scale. You take the selfie from your starting weight and compare it, side by side, with one you take after the first three weeks. If you don't see results, you will reflect on your S.P.E.E.D. profile and change your actions.

SUGAR CRAVINGS DISSIPATE

The first three days when you limit the amount of sugar in your diet are the toughest, but maintaining that action for the next eighteen days gets easier. By the twenty-first day, I promise you that you won't be missing the soda or morning doughnut. You won't be hunting for dessert after dinner, or a piece of candy to pick you up after lunch. In twenty-one days, your taste buds will have regenerated and they will be finding naturally sweet foods like fruit more satisfying than a bag of Skittles.

EXERCISE ADAPTATION

Starting a new exercise regimen isn't easy on the body. You might be sore from strength training, tired from performing cardio, or struggling a little to fit in all of this additional activity. For the first three days it might feel like the mental and physical struggle is unending, but I guarantee you that within the next twenty-one days your body will have adapted to the new stimuli. Gradually the mile that took you 17 minutes to run the first day won't feel overwhelming anymore—you'll probably be running it in closer to 13 minutes! And instead of curling a max weight of 10 pounds, you will now be aiming for 12 pounds. Your lungs will have become more efficient, your muscles will have become stronger, and your mind will have become tougher.

BODY FUNCTIONS EFFICIENTLY

In the past, you may have felt constipated, bloated, fatigued, or lethargic. But after three weeks of eating healthy, drinking water, eliminating sugar, moving your body, and prioritizing sleep, your body will have eliminated the toxins that once weighed down your system. By creating a daily eating, training, digesting, and sleeping routine, your body will be becoming a lean, mean, fat-churning machine!

The Three-Month Rule

Every season has its end, and so do your goals. Aiming to complete three-month intervals will keep you focused and will help you work hard, knowing that you will see a significant and specific transformation in that time.

FIRST SIGNIFICANT TRANSFORMATION

If you saw your first body transformation at just three weeks, imagine quadrupling that time and effort and seeing the results at the end of three months. The transformation after four consecutive three-week cycles will be substantial! In nearly ninety days, you will feel like a new person. Your ability to set a goal and accomplish it will have left an indelible mark on your mentality. Your face and waist will be smaller, your legs will be lighter, and your smile will be bigger. Most important, you will be incredibly proud, having taught yourself a new pattern for success. While you may not yet be at your ultimate weight goal, breaking your journey into three-day, three-week, and three-month sessions makes reaching that destination achievable.

PART 2

S.P.E.E.D.

Set the Goal

Plan the Attack

Envision the Journey

Execute the Plan

Deliver the Results

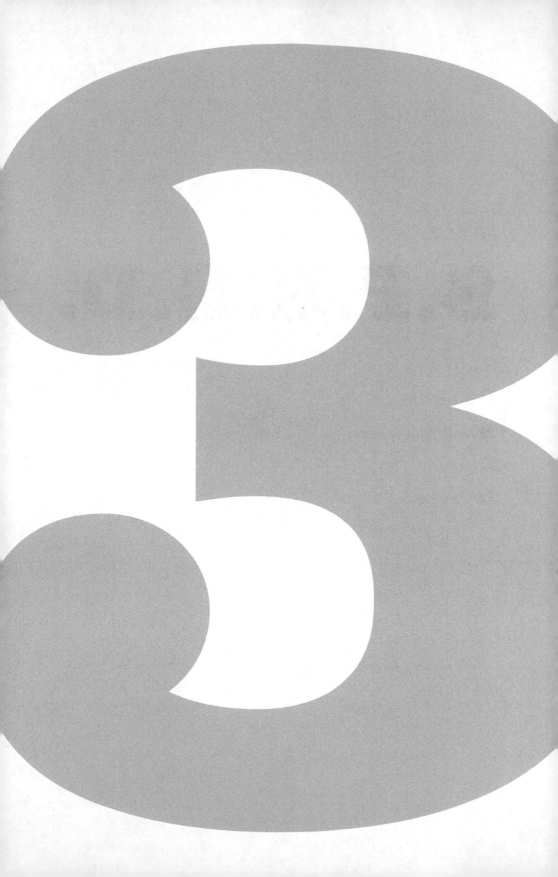

S.P.E.E.D. TOWARD YOUR FIRST GOAL

Right now you are inspired, motivated, and driven. You are at stage one, the S.P.E.E.D. stage. This is an exciting time, when your engine is turned on, when your plane taxis down the runway, and when it takes off to soar into the stratosphere.

You need this momentum. The energy you spend during this first stage will build the S.P.E.E.D. you require to reach success. This early stage is all about **S**etting goals, **P**lanning your attack, **E**nvisioning your journey, **E**xecuting your plan, and **D**elivering the results. The S.P.E.E.D. acronym is an easy way to remember this stage. It's a method that simplifies your approach, intensifies your force, and sharpens your focus. So, start manifesting your dreams by creating a strong desire.

This chapter is for developing the internal rigor that will keep you moving toward your goal. Maintaining your motivation is the magic behind your long-term success. Will there be times of struggle? Yes. Will you make mistakes along the way? Certainly. Does anyone fail on this No More Excuses program? Absolutely not! This plan doesn't start and end in three months; this is an attitude that will carry you far—the rest of your life. If you accept the setbacks as part of this process, you will *not* fail this time.

Imagine your *best body*. Think about how you want to feel, what you want to do, and where you want to go. Envision yourself confidently shopping for sleeveless tops or a form-fitting dress. Picture yourself walking down a beach, hiking up a mountain, or running a 10K. *Really think about it.* Fill your mind with longing for a life of accomplishments, for this incredible effort to build your best body.

S.P.E.E.D. Explained

Let's get started—and let's get there fast! I hear you when it comes to losing weight. It never seems to happen fast enough. And while on any program you will hit plateaus, deal with distractions, and have to bust some excuses, you will get to your goal faster if you use S.P.E.E.D. So, S.P.E.E.D. is a goal-setting model that you will use to effectively and efficiently target your short-term goals.

Too often, people set out to achieve a really ambitious goal without having a clear plan for how to do it. For instance, wanting to look great at an upcoming family event is a great motivator, but you need a strategy for living every day until you've achieved your goal. If you don't break that goal into more manageable pieces, it's going to become overwhelming and you'll find it hard to stick to it.

That's what is so amazing about S.P.E.E.D. It gives you a way to focus on your overall process each day, so that you don't get derailed by the little setbacks that are inevitable in life.

Here's how it works!

SET THE GOAL. Are you competitive? Do you want to impress people? Do you want to look great for an upcoming event? Figure out what your motivation is and write it down as a specific short-term goal to set your sights on. It's not enough to say you want to lose weight and eat healthier. You must desire, dream, and dedicate yourself to a specific goal, in a specific time period. A deadline creates a level of urgency that can motivate you to follow through, despite the challenges you will face after setting that goal.

For example, your goal could be to fit into your favorite pair of jeans, the jeans that have been sitting on the top shelf of your closet because they have been too snug for several years. Or perhaps your goal is to run a 10K race or to perform ten pull-ups. Whatever you choose, create a deadline of exactly three months from today. Write down your goal, and put it somewhere that you will see every day: on the refrigerator, above your computer screen, on the bathroom mirror—any place that will be a daily reminder.

PLAN THE ATTACK. A good plan of action makes even the loftiest goals possible. Once you set your goal, work backward to plan your attack. For example, if you want to lose 25 pounds in three months, you need to lose 8 pounds each month or 2 pounds each week. It takes 3,500 calories to burn 1 pound of body fat, so you need a diet and exercise regimen that will get you burning 7,000 calories each week. Seem like a lot? Not if you create a caloric deficit of 500 calories in your diet for seven days; then you will have burned 3,500 calories in that one week! Your second pound lost will come from consistent exercise. With this knowledge, losing 25 pounds in three months feels more reachable!

If your goal is to run a half-marathon (13.1 miles), start by focusing on running 1 mile, rather than staring down the whole distance at once. Pick a training program and integrate it into your life, one day at a time. As you build strength and endurance, you can add mileage weekly. After a few months of cardio conditioning, a half-marathon will become more mentally feasible, but it starts with running 1 mile today!

Building your best body is 80 percent planning and 20 percent execution. So this is the moment to create a blueprint for what you will build to achieve your goal. There are resources in this book to help you get organized and create a plan that works realistically with your lifestyle; in Chapter 7, you'll find guides for healthier eating, in Chapter 6 and the Appendix, you'll find workout guides that you can customize. Plan a workout schedule and make time to prepare your meals. Give away your junk food and clear out your cupboards of any trigger snacks. Stock your refrigerator with fresh fruits and vegetables. Buy all your necessary equipment, including a water bottle, sweat towels, workout outfits, healthy cookbooks, exercise DVDs, and/or a gym membership. Load your guns and prepare for battle.

ENVISION THE JOURNEY. Visualize the steps you will take to achieve your goal. Some people fail before they begin because they are stuck on bad past experiences. To succeed, envision yourself succeeding. Write down your goals and remind yourself of them daily. When you wake up each day, imagine how your day will go and see yourself saying no to procrastination. Rehearse persuasive arguments against eating poorly. Focus on staying strong and avoiding temptation. When you've fought the battle in your mind, you've gained the mental strength to win the real battles in life.

Picture yourself gathering the ingredients for your next healthy meal, preparing the meal, and enjoying the delicious results. Before you start a workout, visualize yourself warming up, taking the first few steps, and then launching into it. Imagine pushing through your physical discomfort and completing each set with stamina to spare. Think about how good you will feel, how strong you will become, and how happy you will be when you walk out of the gym after a powerful workout. These mental images will keep you motivated, and they will help you to be aware of your goal each day. (Keep in mind that there is a difference between a little discomfort and pain. If you are in serious pain, stop what you are doing and, if necessary, seek a medical professional.)

EXECUTE THE PLAN. Of course, you can't just visualize success—you also need to take action! This means waking up each morning and preparing those meals, completing your training, taking your vitamins, getting enough water, and enjoying a full night's sleep. The simple act of following through on what you *say* you will do is success in itself. Perhaps your action won't be 100 percent perfect, but no one is perfect. Just make it a point to stop procrastinating and start doing what you *say* you're going to do. The more your actions support your plans, the closer you come to achieving your best body.

DELIVER THE RESULTS. Perhaps you've tried other diets before but gave up when you weren't getting the results you wanted. That's not going to happen this time. The No More Excuses diet is not just about celebrating results; it's also about celebrating all the work you put into achieving good health. Each day you have countless opportunities to do something good for yourself. Every bite of fresh food, every half hour of heart-pumping movement, and every good night's sleep are steps toward achieving your goal. Take the time to applaud yourself with each step you take!

Once you seed a desire, that intention will grow daily through attention, reflection, and action. Put aside some time to dream, allowing your thoughts to implant those desires.

Using S.P.E.E.D. to Realize Your Goals: Some Examples

Everyone's short-term goals are different, but the techniques for achieving them are the same. To take focused and deliberate action, you must set, plan, envision, execute, and deliver. Now that you have been given the program rules, you can apply them to any goal and succeed. Here are some examples of how to apply the S.P.E.E.D. strategy.

GOAL: Lose 25 pounds

SET: On your fitness calendar, write down your goal weight of 25 pounds less than what you currently weigh. Consider tracking all areas of progress, including body composition, vitals, and fitness level. For the majority of overweight people, losing 1 to 2 pounds per week is normal and healthy.

PLAN: Make an action plan for how you will lose those pounds. Decide how you will be documenting your daily intake. Mark off the days every two weeks that you will measure your progress. Figure out how many calories you need to create a deficit. Schedule the most realistic times for you to train. Delegate a space where you are going to work out, and purchase any fitness supplies you'll need. Complete your fitness calendar, write down your planned treat meals, and post some motivational quotes. It's time to get serious!

ENVISION: Wake up each day with intention. Envision completing a successful workout, overcoming temptation at a party, or enjoying a guilt-free splurge. Think about the person you want to become, and focus on positive thoughts and progressive actions all day. If you know you've been challenged by waking up early to work out, then picture yourself not hitting the snooze button when your alarm goes off and getting up out of bed without struggling. If you know there will be treats at work or snacks during your children's playtime, envision bringing your own healthy meal and rejecting any food outside your nutrition plan.

EXECUTE: Now that you've set your goal, planned your journey, and envisioned your success, you need to take action. Start eating your healthy breakfast each morning, drinking your water, and exercising four times a week. Write down your food intake. Measure the changes in your body every three weeks. There will be days you will struggle and days you will succeed; just focus on staying on course until your good actions become good habits.

DELIVER: Do not make a decision about your results until you reach the three-week mark. Have you lost 5 pounds? Has your activity level increased? Did your body fat drop 1 to 2 percent? After three weeks, measure your success and reflect on your plan. Look at your food diary and review your fitness calendar. See where you are struggling and identify ways to overcome those struggles. No one is perfect, so don't feel frustrated if you aren't delivering as fast as you planned. Restructure your short-term action plan and start setting achievable goals you can reach.

GOAL: Run your first 5K

SET: Set your goal, which will include a date when your 5K will be completed. Sign up for a race in your area so that you are accountable!

PLAN: Plan your running schedule. If you have no experience running, make your goal to run 1 mile a day, a few times a week. As your endurance builds, you can increase your miles every few weeks; remember, your goal is to feel challenged but not get in over your head. Purchase running shoes with good support and find some running partners who can help and encourage you—someone who has run a 5K race before, a friend who will participate in your training, or a beginner with whom you can share the learning.

ENVISION: Becoming a serious runner is an endeavor that requires consistency, persistence, and belief. Envision yourself moving swiftly and smoothly as you run past houses or along park roads, pushing past physical discomfort and completing your daily mileage. If you can see yourself feeling tired, weak, or incapable, your body will listen to your mind's voice and discourage you; don't allow that to happen. If you are not yet a runner, believe right now that you are! What you think, you will become.

EXECUTE: Start running! Follow your running schedule. Ensure your nutrition reflects your energy requirements, and don't forget to take a breather. Taking action means training, eating, and resting!

DELIVER: Within three weeks your body will have acclimated to your new training habits and your composition, vitals, and fitness levels will have altered. Your body may have dropped some fat, your leg and core muscles will be stronger, your resting heart rate will have declined, and your endurance will have increased. If you are still struggling to follow through, if you are not eating properly or prioritizing your training, then you're definitely not delivering the results you need to hit your 5K goal. Reflect on your progress and restart the S.P.E.E.D. plan by setting shorter, more achievable goals. If you have succeeded at your running goal and are making progress, set a new round of S.P.E.E.D. goals that will take you to the next level.

While the S.P.E.E.D. strategy can be used for many long-term goals, I often use it to set short-term, daily goals. For example, I have a foot injury that prevents me from applying any weight on my right foot right now. So, in accordance with my "excuse," I've created this S.P.E.E.D. strategy:

....

SET: Stay active by connecting with a favorite childhood activity; eat cleaner.

PLAN: Eat five small meals with a 40/30/30 ratio (see Chapter 7), with high emphasis on protein. What will I eat? Where will I get the ingredients? When I was young, I used to love swimming. Perform a core routine (no weight on legs) and swim laps for 30 minutes.

ENVISION: I will pack my swimsuit and towel, and go to the gym after dropping my child off at school. I envision the locker room, the cold water, the people around me. I know I'll be limping, probably nervous about being in a swimsuit, and likely fatigued from this new exercise as a result, but I envision pushing myself to finish in 30 minutes.

EXECUTE: I schedule my meals for 9 AM/12 PM/3 PM/5 PM/8 PM, and I take action! I start with my first meal of the day, then drop my child at school, then head to the gym, then proceed with the rest of my work day, including my planned meals.

DELIVER: At the end of the day, I consider whether I followed through or "failed." The good part is, I didn't really fail—I failed only if I didn't reflect and figure out what prevented me from executing the plan. Did I forget my swimsuit? Was I unmotivated? Did I forget to eat? I reflect and move forward.

Thoughts Become Reality

Even if you don't feel strong, svelte, or sexy right now, believe that ideal version of yourself is just around the corner! When I was 30 pounds overweight, I wrote the phrase "You are strong, fit, and beautiful" in the front of my journal. I didn't really feel this way; I was often battling thoughts of fatigue, frustration, and failure. It's easy to get on the shame train and ride it for a week or more, but keep in mind that this track leads nowhere worth going. When you view the world through a negative lens, you can never see any positive possibilities. In fact, you won't see much at all, because your vision is blocked by images of the things you can't do. So, I repeated positive affirmations about my body, even though in those days my legs felt like tree trunks, my belly looked like gelatin, and my arms shook every time I waved. Those affirmations allowed me to keep believing that it *was possible* to have a body I would love one day, even if I didn't have it at that moment.

Protect your thoughts, because what you believe is what you will become. The first belief you must have in this journey is that you will complete it. You *can* do this. When you truly commit to the journey, you redefine your purpose and reshape your identity.

When you live a purposeful life, you develop a passion for living, a resilient attitude that only gets stronger, even in times of stress. Some of your purpose stems from desire, but most of it comes from pressure.

USING S.P.E.E.D. TO SET YOUR GOALS

1 **Find some paper and write down your goals.** Choose at least five goals that are specific: "I want to fit into old jeans," "I will lose 20 pounds," or "I'm running a 5K." The goals should be well defined and segmented into units that are manageable. Tape your goals to your bathroom mirror, so that you will be able to see them often.

2 **Invest in your End Date.** What will you do to motivate you to stay on track so you reach your three-month date? You invest in something that will make a personal connection with that date. Is there a family event that you can orient toward? A birthday coming up? Can you schedule a special trip or activity? If you want to add pressure to your weight-loss journey, create a level of social accountability by telling others of your goal and lifestyle change. By revealing your intention, you start to align with people who are on the same journey and you deflect people who don't bring value to your life. Being around people with healthier habits will encourage you to persist in social situations when there's pressure to eat poorly.

3 **Measure your starting point.** Remember, progress is made when progress is measured. Get on a scale, and do not be afraid of the number because that is just your starting point. Put that number in your journal. Use a measuring tape to measure your neck, shoulders, arms, chest, waist, hips, legs, and calves. Make sure you know exactly where you placed the tape by keeping notes in your journal. If you have access to a trainer at the gym, have the person take your body fat via skin calipers. (If you can't, that's okay; it's just another measurement to track your progress.) I say more about why this measuring is so important in Chapter 4, but in short, you can't celebrate how far you've come if you don't know where you started!

4 **Perform a series of fitness tests.** In Chapter 6, I give you a list of exercises that can test your fitness: How many military push-ups can you do without dropping? How long can you perform a plank? How fast can you run a mile? Put your results in your journal.

5 **Write down everything you're eating.** It's key to see your eating patterns: When do you eat, what do you eat, or why do you eat (or overeat!)? In Chapter 7, I give you my rules for a healthy diet, which you will be able to customize to fit your needs.

6 **Create a fitness calendar.** This large poster-like three-month calendar will keep you accountable and record your workout progress. You can color-code it as you complete your workouts, but do not write down your workouts in advance—only record them once you've completed them. Write down your goals, your power words, and your important event dates.

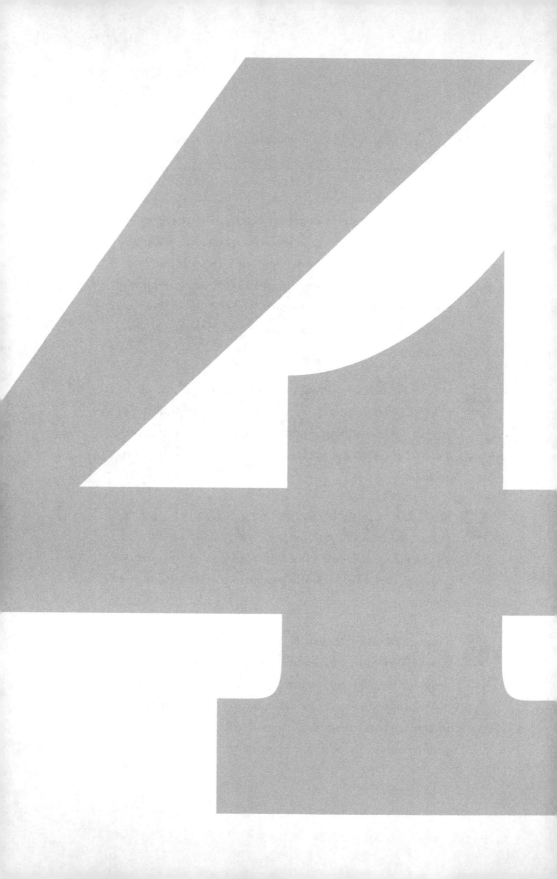

GET READY! GET SET! GO!

As I said in the last chapter, it's important to start your No More Excuses journey with an honest assessment of where you currently are. To calculate your success, you need to be able to measure your progress.

This is a good time to check with your doctor before proceeding with any diet or exercise plan. After you get the go-ahead, begin measuring your baseline. Most people define how healthy they are by how much they weigh; however, how healthy you are really depends on several different variables. You should, at this beginning point, measure three indicators of your overall health: your body composition, your vital statistics, and your fitness level. I show you how to measure each of these so that you can compare these baseline figures with the recommended averages and document your progress in your journal. No matter what the numbers say right now, don't be discouraged: This is about finding out where you are today so you can develop a safe and effective program to get where you want to go.

Your Body Composition

This is what you can externally see. You can easily assess your physical progress through your weight, body circumference, and clothing size, making it the most common measurement people use to assess their health.

BODY MASS INDEX (BMI)

The most popular and controversial test that physicians have used is the body mass index (BMI). This is a mathematical formula that takes into account both height and weight. The BMI equals a person's weight in kilograms divided by his or her height in meters squared (BMI = kg/m^2). To convert your pounds into kilograms, simply divide your weight by 2.2. For example, if you weigh 150 pounds, your conversion weight is 68.2 kilograms. If your BMI measures 18.5 to 24.9, you are considered of normal weight; anything more is considered overweight or obese.

The BMI is not always the best reflection of how healthy you are, however. While this test is widely used, athletes could be cited as overweight because they have extra muscle. That's why it's important to utilize several different tests to determine your level of health. If you have more muscle and rank higher on the BMI chart (see page 41), don't be discouraged. We will review several body and fitness tests that measure your starting point.

BODY FAT

Measuring your body fat is another important tool to see how much of your weight consists of pure fat versus solid muscle. There are two types of fat. Subcutaneous fat is the common fat found beneath the skin. Visceral fat, a more dangerous fat, is hidden in between your organs and is stored deep within your abdomen. Too much

BODY MASS INDEX (BMI) FOR ADULTS

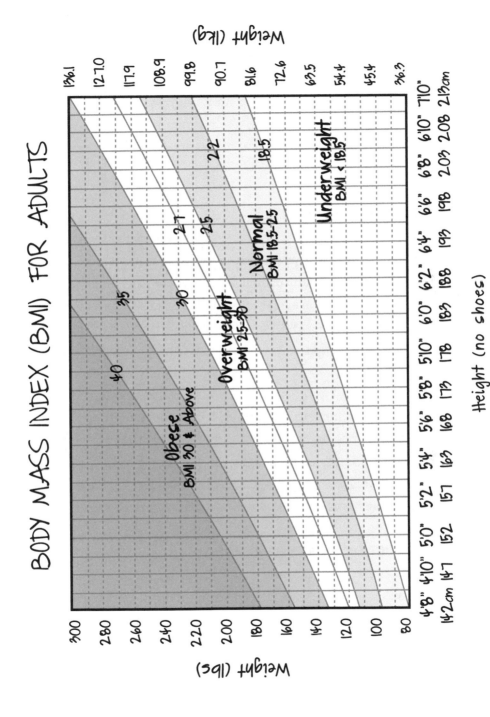

Weight (kg)

196.1 127.0 117.9 108.9 99.8 90.7 81.6 72.6 63.5 54.4 45.4 36.3

4'8" 4'10" 5'0" 5'2" 5'4" 5'6" 5'8" 5'10" 6'0" 6'2" 6'4" 6'6" 6'8" 6'10" 7'10"
142cm 147 152 157 163 168 173 178 183 188 193 198 203 208 213cm

Height (no shoes)

Obese
BMI 30 & Above

Overweight
BMI 25-30

Normal
BMI 18.5-25

Underweight
BMI < 18.5

40   35   30   27   25   22   18.5

Weight (lbs)

300 280 260 240 220 200 180 160 140 120 100 80

body fat is linked to high levels of "bad" cholesterol, hypertension, diabetes, stroke, and heart disease.

Only a professional with proper equipment can accurately measure your body fat. Many gyms will have someone on hand to do this without much cost. For a male adult, an average amount of body fat is 18 to 24 percent. For a female adult, it's 25 to 31 percent. If you don't belong to a gym, search for centers in your area that can test your body fat.

WAIST-TO-HIP RATIO

Once you know your BMI and percentage of body fat, the last thing you should measure is your waist-to-hip ratio. You can probably take a good look at your body shape and see where your fat is stored. To determine if you have a healthy waist-to-hip ratio, use a measuring tape to measure the smallest part of your waist, usually just above the belly button. Then measure the widest part of your hips, which will include part of your buttocks. Divide your waist measurement by your hip measurement to find your ratio. Research shows that women with a waist-to-hip ratio of 0.80 or below and men with a ratio of 0.95 or below face fewer health risks. In other words, storing excessive fat in the abdominal region (aka apple-shaped bodies) is linked to weight-related diseases like diabetes, heart disease, and lower kidney function.

OTHER BODY MEASUREMENTS

Since a pound of fat is three times larger than a pound of muscle, you could be gaining weight but losing inches. Check your body measurements once a month to document your progress. With a soft measuring tape, measure your neck, shoulders, biceps, chest, waist, hips, upper/middle/lower thighs, and calves. There is no standard for these measurements, but the numbers will help you measure your physical progress without a scale.

Your Vital Statistics

The "vitals" are your internal measurements of progress. Most often, the changes your body will undergo are areas you won't see in a mirror. Through exercise and good nutrition, though, you will improve your body's "motor." Your lungs will hold more oxygen, your organs will more efficiently process foods, and your blood will flow more effortlessly through your body. By checking your starting "vitals," you'll be able to measure the results of your journey and see your numbers improve in just one month's time.

BLOOD PRESSURE

Of the two major ways that doctors assess the immediate health of your heart, blood pressure represents the amount of pressure your circulating blood is exerting against the sides of your blood vessels. To measure your blood pressure, you can use a sphygmomanometer found at most pharmacies or in a doctor's office. You can also purchase an affordable blood pressure kit from major retail stores. Normal blood pressure ranges from 110 to 150 millimeters (as the heart beats) over 60 to 80 millimeters (as the heart rests between beats). For young adults, a blood pressure of 120/80 indicates your heart is healthy (150/90 for 60 and above). If your numbers are higher, this is an indication of hypertension, or high blood pressure, which can lead to heart disease.

PULSE, OR HEART RATE

Besides your blood pressure, your pulse is an important measure of your heart health. Particularly, your pulse shows how hard your heart is working, either at rest or during activity. To measure your pulse, find the radial artery along the side of your neck, or at your wrist on the thumb side, and count how many pulses you feel in a minute. An average person's pulse measures 60 to 80 beats per minute at rest, although an athlete's pulse can be as low as between 35 and 50 beats. The best time to measure your resting pulse is when you wake up in the morning, before performing any activity. Lie in bed, set your timer, and count how many times your heart beats per minute. A good trick is to measure your heartbeat for 15 seconds and multiply that number by 4. As your health improves, you will notice your resting heart rate decline, indicating that your heart isn't working as hard.

BLOOD SUGAR

Controlling your blood sugar/glucose levels through exercise and diet will help protect you from developing type 2 diabetes and the complications that go with it, like kidney failure, heart disease, blindness, and lower-limb amputation. You can measure your blood sugar with a portable electronic device or at your physician's office. A healthy blood sugar range is between 70 and 100 mg/dL and can rise to 140 mg/dL after eating. A friend of mine was diagnosed as pre-diabetic when his blood sugar levels hovered around 170 after eating. He cut down on his sugar intake and began walking regularly, which brought his blood sugar levels down to a healthy range.

Your Overall Fitness Level

Any judgment of fitness focuses on function. That is, what your body is capable of doing. It's a measurement that bridges the gap between how your body looks and how it operates. Fitness includes flexibility, cardio fitness, and strength.

FLEXIBILITY

To measure your lower back and hamstring flexibility, simply get a sit-and-reach box (available in sports shops and online) or sit on the floor with your shoes off, legs shoulder-width apart and extended straight out. Tape a ruler on the ground between your feet, extending away from you. Place your hands on top of each other, palms facing down and slowly reach forward toward your toes. After making three practice reaches, hold the fourth reach for at least 2 seconds and notice where on the ruler you've reached. An adult male with excellent flexibility can reach anywhere between 6.5 and 10.5 inches beyond his toes. An adult female with excellent flexibility can reach anywhere between 8 and 11.5 inches.

If you don't want to go through the hassle of finding a sit-and-reach box or a ruler, just take a cellphone picture of how far you can stretch. Sit straight in a straddle stretch, with knees slightly bent, and reach for your toes as far as you can. Have someone snap your farthest reach and date your picture.

#NSV

NSV stands for "Non-Scale Victory." Too often we measure our progress solely based on what the scale says. I encourage you to discover your #NSV in your fitness journey. Your success is dependent on how good you feel, how consistent you are with the program, and how healthy you become. If you can run longer, lift heavier, fit into old clothes, overcome sugar cravings, run a 5K, or confidently wear a bikini—then it's a victory!

CARDIO FITNESS

To measure your cardio fitness, hop on a treadmill or go outside and start running. Time how long it takes you to complete 1 mile at a good jog. When you finish, record the time and your heart rate. As your heart health improves, you will build strength and endurance.

Another way to test your cardio health is to get a 12-inch-high bench or box and step on and off the box for 3 minutes. This is a basic step test that involves enduring physical demand on your heart. After 3 minutes, remain standing and immediately check your pulse. If you are a man and your pulse is below 85 beats per minute, you have excellent cardiovascular fitness. If you are a woman with a pulse below 92 beats per minute, you are in rocking good shape. Everybody else? Now you have an idea what to strive for!

STRENGTH

One of the basic tests of fitness includes no equipment at all. Push-ups are a great upper-body exercise that uses your chest, shoulders, triceps, and core. To perform a full push-up test, you warm up with some stretching and light activity. Then, you position your body facedown on the floor, legs extended straight back and toes bent, hands shoulder-width apart with elbows straight and arms fully extended. While keeping a straight line from your toes to your hips and to the shoulders, you lower your upper body so your elbows bend to 90 degrees. Then, you raise your body to the earlier position and count this as one rep. You continue raising and lowering, and complete as many repetitions as possible without breaking form.

While performing full push-ups, you lift nearly 75 percent of your total body weight; if you do a modified push-up (knees bent, holding some of your weight), you lift about 60 percent. Both types of push-up are fine as long as you challenge yourself. Record the total number of push-ups completed. If you are a fit adult male between the ages of 20 and 40, performing 50 or more push-ups is considered excellent. If you are a fit adult female between 20 and 40 years old, performing 30 or more push-ups is considered above average. However, if you are a beginner, performing just 5 to 10 push-ups (or none at all!) for both men and women is normal. Keep in mind that this is a test, and the goal is to become stronger in the weeks to come.

Another good test of strength is the plank hold. Get into a push-up position with your toes and forearms on the floor. Keep a neutral spine and hips squared and draw in your belly button toward the small of your back. Use a timer and measure how long you can hold the plank position.

Building your best body means serious business, so you need to record your reps to establish your baseline. From this day forward, your goal will be to shift these numbers in your desired direction. Remember, the direction of your journey depends on the actions you take, because every action has a consequence. You will start to see this incredible power that you have to control these consequences when you take proper action today.

Your Nutritional Baseline

In addition to documenting your physical starting point, it's time to establish your nutritional baseline. For the next three days, you won't focus on dieting; you'll eat as your normally do, but you'll write everything down. For each meal or snack, you'll record the time, meal, portion size, and calorie count. Just make sure you are documenting everything you eat: the bite from your child's sandwich, the piece of chocolate you took from your coworker's desk, the sweetened tea you drank during lunch. This exercise not only creates awareness of what you are consuming but it also holds you accountable. After you write down your intake, you will assess the results and seek areas where you can cut portion sizes, add a healthy meal, or skip an empty-calorie dessert.

Setting yourself up for success isn't just about throwing out the junk food and joining a gym; it's also about setting balanced goals, creating a support network, and developing ways to stay

ACTION CALENDAR

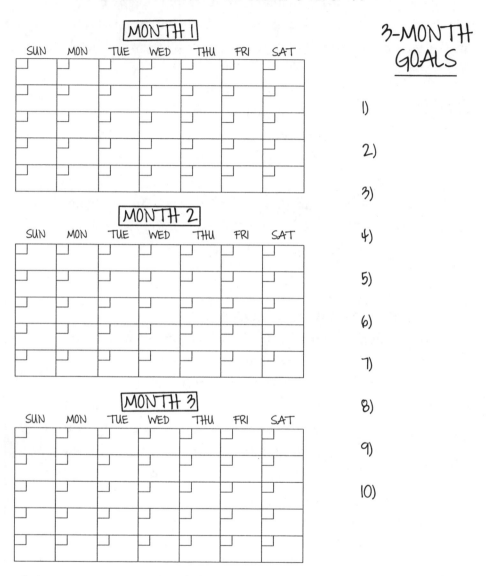

MONTH 1

SUN	MON	TUE	WED	THU	FRI	SAT

MONTH 2

SUN	MON	TUE	WED	THU	FRI	SAT

MONTH 3

SUN	MON	TUE	WED	THU	FRI	SAT

3-MONTH GOALS

1)

2)

3)

4)

5)

6)

7)

8)

9)

10)

PATIENCE · CONSISTENCY · FOCUS · FAITH

PROGRESS CHART

	WEEK 1	WEEK 3	WEEK 6	WEEK 9	WEEK 12
DATE					
WEIGHT					
BMI					
BODY FAT%					
WAIST-TO-HIP RATIO					
RESTING HEART RATE					
NECK					
SHOULDERS					
BICEPS					
CHEST					
WAIST					
HIPS					
THIGHS					
UPPER					
MIDDLE					
LOWER					
CALVES					
BLOOD PRESSURE					
BLOOD SUGAR					
FLEXIBILITY					
MILE TIME					
STEP TEST					
MAX PUSH-UPS					
PLANK HOLD					

accountable. If you try to make a change that only impacts one aspect of your life, you will eventually falter. This program isn't about taking a break from your real life until you shed enough pounds; it's about making positive changes to your life as a whole, so that you can perform at your peak level all the time. So, as you set your goals, think about how they are going to impact the rest of your life and what you might need to change in order for that to happen.

Now that you've got your physical baselines, have observed your current diet, have assembled your fitness tools, and have established your goals, it's time to take intentional action. This journey is about making no excuses; it's about focusing on reflection, preparation, action, and execution.

So, let's go!

CREATE A THREE-MONTH ACCOUNTABILITY BOARD

One of the most effective actions I have taken has been to create a three-month fitness calendar. Since I don't work with a trainer, it was important to keep track of my training days; it is also a great visual to keep me on track. Every time I trained, I wrote down what exercises I performed and which muscles I worked. This record keeping kept the emphasis on process, rather than results. If you notice there are many blank squares in your calendar, it immediately tells you that you're falling behind.

Here's what you need to do:

1. Print out three blank monthly calendars and paste them side by side on a large poster board.

2. Place the calendar where you will see it every day.

3. Write your goals on the poster, including six things you will focus on in the next three months.

4. Each day, write down what training you did and put a big X on your rest days.

5. Utilize the calendar to record how much you weigh each week and when you had your splurges. If you are a woman, indicate your menstrual cycle, as you will notice patterns around this time.

6. Use highlighters, colored pens, or particular shapes to make the calendar more graphically colorful. For example, I use green to indicate running days, red for rest days.

7. Add inspirational or motivational words, people's pictures, and catchphrases on the poster.

8. Don't let more than three days go by without updating your calendar. You will forget what you did.

9. Review the calendar weekly. Adjust your training goals to make them achievable.

THE NO MORE EXCUSES RULES

So you have your goal, you're fired up, and you're ready to go. Now what? In this chapter I lay out the nine steps of the program that you will use to achieve your S.P.E.E.D. goal. Later in the book, I go into more detail about your workouts, but this chapter describes the overall techniques for customizing the plan to fit your body's needs.

A healthy person practices healthy habits. This program focuses on changing your habits to include actions that will speed up your metabolism, detox your system, strengthen your body, and balance your blood sugar. Your good habits will create actions that will lead to your success.

Everyone has individual, short-term goals. This program is designed to provide a basic execution plan with core guidelines that are flexible for reaching your personal goals. If your goal is to lose weight, gain muscle, become a better runner, tighten up your tummy, or build bigger biceps, you can use the S.P.E.E.D. method and these rules to reach that goal. Keep in mind that you are your best advocate when you're designing a diet and exercise regimen. Discovering your mental, emotional, and physical strengths and weaknesses is all part of this No More Excuses process. You will find out what works best for you only if you are willing to try things that may end up not working; the faster you fail, the faster you'll find the techniques that succeed!

You deserve to have a body that you love. If you don't yet have one that you love, then you need to believe in and take this No More Excuses journey. This is a new route, marked on a road map that's easier to follow. You aren't fast-climbing this weight-loss mountain so you can overheat and exhaust your engine; you are going up the mountain slowly, making gradual changes and developing strengths that will move you past each plateau.

Throughout the book, I give you strategies and suggestions for how to eat, exercise, and evaluate your progress, but those are also the basic principles of the program! There is a tried-and-true way of losing weight and of speeding up your metabolism, and these rules embody that method. While these rules might seem simple, they are game-changing life lessons when you use them properly. Let's look at each of them in more detail.

1. EAT BREAKFAST EVERY MORNING. After a full night's rest, your body wakes in a fasted state; you have to wake up your metabolism as well so that your body's engine is revved up for the day's activities. It's important to refuel with a healthy meal, even though you may not feel hungry. Eating a solid breakfast will also mean you will not overeat during lunch.

Many people think that in order to lose weight, they have to stop eating. Wrong! If your metabolism receives food on a steady

PROGRAM RULES

1. Eat breakfast every morning.

2. Write down everything you eat.

3. Work out three to five times a week.

4. Drink only water, including an optional 2 to 3 cups of black coffee or unsweetened tea each day.

5. Eat small meals containing protein, healthy fats, and carbohydrates throughout the day.

6. Plan your treat meals, which you can have in moderation.

7. Stop eating three hours before bedtime.

8. Measure yourself every three weeks.

9. Reflect on your program weekly.

basis, then it will speed up, but if the body's food supply is intermittent, then the metabolism will slow down, storing food as reserves. You need your body to trust that you will feed it regularly, and a great way to establish that trust is with breakfast each morning. The goal is to build a lean, mean fat-burning machine. I'm not suggesting you have a giant stack of pancakes and orange juice every morning, though. Start your day with a boost of nutrients that leave you feeling energized and poised to excel.

I often eat breakfast on the go! Here are some of my favorite morning meals:

Egg white omelet with a small bowl of oatmeal on the side

Cottage cheese with fruit

Banana and almonds

Breakfast burrito: 2 egg whites, 1 whole egg, spinach, and low-fat cheese in a spinach wrap

Fruit smoothie: ½ cup strawberries, ½ cup blueberries, ½ banana, handful of spinach, and 1 cup almond milk

Hunger is a habit; if you've trained your body to starve each morning, you will initially struggle with incorporating a morning meal. Set a goal for yourself to eat breakfast for three consecutive days, and this new habit will become easier. By the end of this program you will have created a whole new body routine, in which you're eating, sleeping, and pooping (yes, I just said that) at the same time each day.

Did you know that 70 percent of your immune system resides in the digestive tract? Cleansing your body daily of waste and toxins helps promote overall well-being. If you don't have a bowel movement every day, then it's time you start looking at your diet and lifestyle.

1. Drink 64 ounces (8 cups) of water daily.

2. Eat three or four servings of raw fruits and vegetables each day.

3. Consume 30 grams of fiber daily.

4. Practice meditation and relaxation techniques like yoga or prayer.

2. WRITE DOWN EVERYTHING YOU EAT. Accountability will prevent you from overeating and will give you a good idea of what you're doing right and wrong. Writing down your foods will allow you to look back and fix areas that need improvement, especially when you hit weight-loss plateaus. Make sure you document the time, portion size, and estimated number of calories. Your diet will be responsible for 80 percent of your results, so it's important to document your food intake.

Use your hand as a general guide for portion size. One serving of protein is a palm-size portion. One serving of carbohydrates is a fist-size portion. Since unsaturated fats are denser and higher in calories, you want to consume a thumb-size portion.

Counting calories will require some homework on your part, but it gets easier with practice. Utilize an online calorie calculator/pocketbook to research calories in your foods. The No More Excuses diet calls for similar foods weekly, so you'll soon become an expert at judging caloric content.

If you see that there are tempting foods you tend to overeat, get rid of them! Nobody needs them there, not even your kids—no matter how much they protest at first. Get organized, plan your grocery list, prepare your meals, and keep healthy snacks in your car, at your office, and in your purse.

3. WORK OUT THREE TO FIVE TIMES A WEEK. Exercise sometimes gets a bad rap—it can take too long, make you uncomfortable, leave you sweaty—but that thinking has got to change! Exercise is a gift you give your body and your mind; it is your fountain of youth, your life's game changer, and your most powerful weight-loss weapon. It will not only rev up your metabolism but also increase its at-rest burn rate. Besides building muscle and protecting your bones, exercise also releases endorphins, a happy hormone that makes you feel less stressed and anxious. Devote 30 to 60 minutes a day three or four times a week (or more) at any exercise that focuses on flexibility, cardio conditioning, and strength training. You need all three components to build a balanced body.

Dedicating 30 minutes a day to moving your body takes only 2 percent of your total day. You can fit this in when you wake up in the morning, during your lunch break, while watching your kids at the park, or right after they fall asleep. Finding the time to exercise will make you more efficient at completing tasks, prioritizing your to-do list, and sacrificing unimportant activities.

4. DRINK ONLY WATER. Oftentimes we consume extra calories in the form of fancy coffee drinks, juices, smoothies, sodas, energy drinks, and sweetened teas. You can eliminate these calories and detox your digestive system simply by drinking only water. Diet sodas and beverages with artificial sugars are not allowed in this program. A Yale University study showed that consuming artificial sweeteners makes you crave sweeteners more; they also cause bloating and digestive issues, so it's best to stay away from them and cleanse your body of toxins.

For the next three weeks, drink only water. You can also have 2 or 3 cups of black coffee or unsweetened tea per day. If you want to add flavoring, put some lemon or thinly cut fruit, mint, or cucumbers in the water. The acidity in lemons helps balance and detoxify your body. You may also indulge in one glass of wine a week, but outside of that, avoid the empty calories in alcohol, as that will slow down your weight-loss progress.

5. EAT SMALL MEALS CONTAINING PROTEIN, HEALTHY FATS, AND CARBOHYDRATES THROUGHOUT THE DAY. Consume 30 percent protein, 30 percent carbohydrates, and 30 percent fats.

You can customize the last 10 percent to reflect your activity level and your short-term goals. Remember that each macronutrient serves a bodily function, so alter your intake depending on what functions your body is performing. For example, if your body requires more energy, it will need more carbohydrates; utilize the flexible 10 percent to carbo-load if you have an intense training schedule. More sedentary individuals might use that 10 percent for additional lean protein or healthy fats. If you ate well during the day and have allotted calories left over for a small splurge, enjoy a miniature chocolate bar or a small portion of your favorite snack. Splurges are allowed (more on this later).

This is not a starvation diet. It's important to consistently fuel your body throughout the day with a balanced menu of whole, unprocessed foods. Don't omit any of your essential macronutrients, as you need protein for muscle building, carbohydrates for energy, and fat for brain health. Eating small meals will keep your blood sugar levels stable and will minimize your chances of overeating.

Dieting is a progression. For example, you can't expect to run a marathon without spending weeks or months training for it, and you can't expect to overhaul your diet overnight. Like training to run a marathon, the diet starts slowly and makes small adjustments until you have established lifelong good habits. You need to build your mental discipline and physical strength to lose weight. If you weigh 200 pounds, you are eating an average of 3,500 calories daily, but starting immediately on a 1,200-calorie/day diet will doom you to failure. Your next weight-loss stop should be to eat like a 190-pound person, cutting down your total calories slowly. Start by consuming 3,000 calories a day and watch your body change. Change always begets change, and at each diet plateau you reach, you can lower your caloric intake or alter your proportion of macronutrients.

6. PLAN YOUR TREAT MEALS, WHICH YOU CAN HAVE IN MODERATION. If you follow a strict 30/30/30 diet plan, then the remaining 10 percent can be used for a light, planned splurge. A splurge is when you consume something outside of your normal diet. For example, since I am a busy working mother, moderation is my mantra. Normally my daily 10 percent (of my total daily intake) is used to eat the leftovers of my child's meal or a square of dark chocolate. However, if I have eaten well all week, without any treats, I top off the week with a satisfying portion of chocolate cake! It's up to you to apply the 10 percent to either daily intake or weekly intake.

Planned treat meals are different from unplanned ones because you *own* your action and you understand why it's important for your overall plan. Most diets fail because they don't leave room for change and, most of all, for balance. Being able to moderately splurge is my saving grace and will become yours also! When you treat yourself to a favorite not-so-healthy dish once in a while, it not only gives you mental satisfaction but it also surprises your body. And surprising your body improves your metabolism because it breaks the pattern of caloric deficit. A treat meal speeds up your metabolism and therefore speeds up the rate of weight loss.

However, a meal only works if you get right back on track immediately after it. There is no guilt involved, so don't skip the next meals, overexercise to compensate, or beat yourself up for allowing that indulgence.

7. STOP EATING THREE HOURS BEFORE BEDTIME. I say stop eating before bedtime for a few reasons. First, there's a lot of late-night snacking for many folks, especially in front of the TV. This can lead to mindless eating and taking in calories that you not only don't need but also aren't even enjoying consuming. If you stop eating after dinner, you're less likely to plow through a quart of ice cream or a bag of chips while watching your favorite show. Also, you're giving your digestive system a solid break from processing foods, the welcome overnight fast that's broken with breakfast the next day. As your body prepares for slumber, you become less active, requiring fewer calories. If you consume a lot of calories at this point and overcompensate for your body's caloric expenditure, those extra calories turn into stored fat.

8. MEASURE YOURSELF EVERY THREE WEEKS. A number on a scale is not the only measure of progress! That's why I want you to perform the measurement tests I describe in Chapter 4 every three weeks. I guarantee that you will see and feel a change; maybe you'll be able to do more push-ups or get closer to touching your toes. Rather than be fixated on just one measure of success, you will appreciate the steady progress that your whole body is making with the good work you're doing every single day.

9. REFLECT ON YOUR PROGRAM WEEKLY. It's important to take time each day to review and consider what you want out of this life. Dreaming of possibilities each day will keep you motivated and focused on the end result. Reflect on your past excuses. Were they that you lacked time to change your life? You didn't have any support? You were under stress? For many people, the resounding reason they don't fulfill their fitness goals is, in truth, that they lack motivation.

So, rather than fall victim to this, write down motivational quotes that will help you make better choices. Post them where you'll see them regularly; for example, I have posted "Focus on Progress, Not Perfection" on my bedroom wall. I've put "Take Action" above my TV, and I have "Nothing Tastes Better Than Being Fit" on my refrigerator. Find quotes and role models that motivate and inspire you, and record them in your journal.

Not only does reflection help you define areas for improvement, but it also helps you document your progress and internal outlook. This journey is not just about attaining physical fitness; it's about learning about you—what makes you motivated, weak, depressed, sad, excited, and, ultimately, successful.

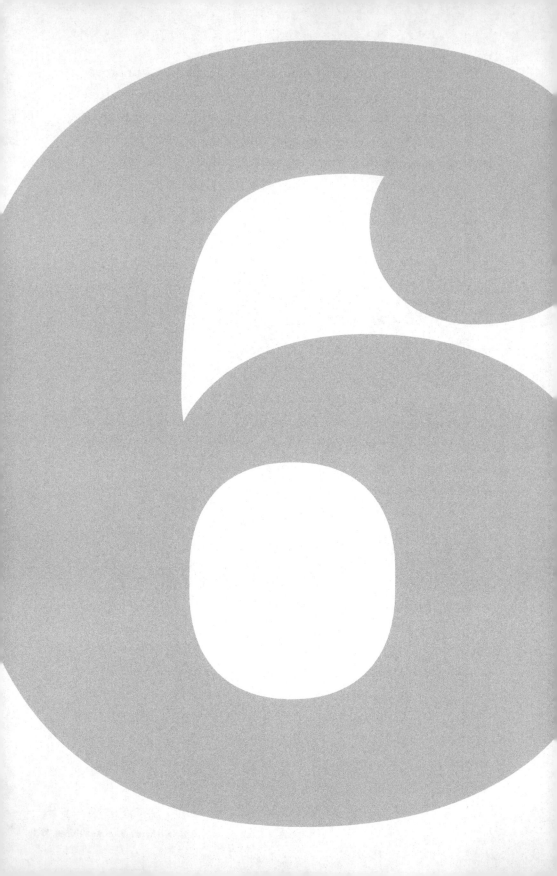

TAKE ACTION

This chapter is where you design the No More Excuses three-week workout program that will challenge your body and yet be suited to your needs. Your workout will fit your schedule and match your strengths. Since a body constantly adapts to external stimuli, you will alter this program every few weeks to prevent getting stuck on plateaus. So, expect to change your fitness program four times in the next three months.

There are three things you need to focus on when creating a complete workout program: strength, cardio, and flexibility. You may excel in one or two, but to have a balanced program, you should incorporate all three. Critically important to developing your skills in each of these areas is *core training*.

Strength helps build metabolism-speeding muscle. Building muscle protects your bones and molds your physique to be lean and toned. Cardio enhances your heart health, increases your endurance, and burns fat. The third component, flexibility, keeps your body agile and nimble. Not only does routine stretching prevent injury and relieve back pain but it also improves your circulation and reduces stress.

Exercises for these components can happen any time, any place, with any movement that is active. You don't have to be in a gym, on a treadmill, or performing the latest fitness craze to see results. You just need strong intention. Be purposeful in waking each day with the specific goal of getting out of your physical comfort zone for at least 20 minutes. The only way to grow is to be challenged. So prepare to work for your best body and get excited about how awesome it's going to feel when you start seeing results. That's why it's called a "workout."

Depending on your mood and motivation, some days will be easier than others. Dance class, for example, rarely feels like work to me—it gets my blood pumping and my lungs gasping for oxygen, so I know my body is being put through the ringer—and I can do it while having fun. I also include some running in my weekly workouts because I've always found running to be challenging. When I run, there are additional benefits because my entire body is engaged and I am mentally forced to pay attention to my breath, my steps, and my motion. I love dance and I hate running. However, I do both because, in order to get results, I need exercise that keeps me motivated but challenged.

While finding the fun factor is important for long-term success, challenging yourself to do something you don't like will move you much farther ahead. There is a difference between moving your body and challenging your body. For example, I'm not a big fan of body weight exercises. I find push-ups, pull-ups, and weighted squats to be incredibly difficult. Although these strength moves often make me feel weak and inept, the mental and physical achievement feels amazing, especially when I break my personal record. Not only am I stronger when I perform these exercises but my body is also more responsive. Having a program of things I enjoy, like dance classes and circuit training, mixed with things I loathe, like body weight exercises, running, and yoga, gets me closer to meeting my physical goals.

The challenge in developing your best body is in incorporating movement whenever you can and training your body so it functions more efficiently. When you perform a cardiovascular activity like running or dancing, you are inhaling oxygen, expanding your lung capacity, challenging your heart, and moving blood through your body so it can provide you with the energy you need to perform that activity. Indeed, your body will look for energy either from the foods you consume (glycogen) or the fat cells in your body. Providing your body with the exact amount of fuel it needs while also maximizing its fat-burning potential takes proper programming.

GET COMFORTABLE WITH BEING UNCOMFORTABLE

The only way to grow is to be challenged, and that includes performing cardio exercise. While dance class is fun, it's definitely harder when I squat lower or make my moves bigger. Get uncomfortable! I used to be a group exercise junkie, but now if I want to really lose weight I get on a treadmill because running is more challenging for me. I use a stair-climber more than an elliptical and an arc trainer more than a stationary bike. You get my drift? Usually, what you hate doing is what's harder for you, but what's harder for you means losing more weight by doing it!

At the end of this chapter you'll find a sampling of balanced workouts that will help you strengthen your core and develop your strength, cardio, and flexibility. But it's important to understand why it all matters!

The Core of Your Workouts

If you want to build an amazing house, you need plans for building it. When you are organized and have all the materials you need, the first thing you do is lay a strong foundation. For exercise, your foundation is your body's core, a powerful place that emits balance, stability, and strength. As you begin to develop, grow, and improve your body, you will be applying cardiovascular and muscular pressure that will improve your physique. While the external pressures placed on your body will cause stress and tension, if your core is strong it will endure these pressures and changes.

Change is the essence of your fitness program; your success relies on how your body strives in the midst of constant change. The basis of your physical improvement is to test how much your body can endure without losing its balance. Each week you will challenge how much weight you can lift before losing form or how long you can hold a yoga pose before falling down.

All these physical abilities are dependent on the strength of your body's core. You must be able to move without losing stability. The more weight you can move with, the more stable you will become. This is where the importance of core comes in.

Imagine a large tree. It has a heavy trunk and various branches that reach up into the sky! Some branches, though, are shorter, skinnier, and sometimes bend sideways. Depending on the environment where it grows, as well as the other trees that surround it, that tree can take any shape or size.

Your body is like a tree. Your core, which comprises your lower back and abdominal regions, is your trunk. Your arms are your branches, and your legs are your roots. Depending on the challenges your environment imposes upon you, your body will either break or grow stronger. You will notice that a tree can grow to great heights if it has nourishment and good soil in which to grow. Your core is the trunk from which all your physical power originates. If you are injured, weak, or imbalanced in your core, your success or growth will be limited.

Some Core Truths

One of the most desirable parts of a human body is a tight, toned midsection. Your core is not just the visual rectus abdominus, which is the six-pack we often see on fitness magazine covers. Your core is also your transverse abdominals, internal and external obliques, and your lower back region. There are a lot of misconceptions about core training, and I don't want you to waste time training in a way that will not be effective for you. Many people focus mainly on the abdominals they can see, but your body's strength is much deeper than those six muscles in the front of your body. The deeper transverse abdominal muscles and their opposing back muscles make up the powerful trunk of your body. If you want to construct a beautiful body, you need that set of muscles.

Core Truth #1: The first step to improving your core is to improve your posture.

When you stand with correct posture, your entire body is in alignment. Your back is straight, chest up, shoulders squared, chin up, and stomach in. Since we live in a more sedentary society, you will notice several posture deviations, including a forward head, a hunched back, forward shoulders/hips, and pronated feet (toes pointing outward). If you have any of these issues, you will need to correct them by stretching tight muscles and strengthening weak muscles. I provide a posture quiz and stretches on pages 236–45.

It is impossible to build a lean tummy if your body is not in alignment. Not only do postural deviations lead to potential injury, but also imbalanced muscles deactivate your core region and prevent you from developing a strong midsection. Oftentimes, achieving stronger abdominals is as simple as standing up taller.

Core Truth #2: Most people who have great abs don't train them all the time.
If you look at the bodies of athletes, they have naturally developed abdominal areas. But here's the secret: Most people who have great abs don't train them all the time. They don't need to because they engage their core when they're kicking a soccer ball, swinging a bat, balancing upright on a bike, or any other activity they're performing.

You don't have to train your abs every day because you are already working them every day! You just need to start engaging them more often. You engage them by challenging your core ever so slightly, whether it's by sitting up straight in a chair and sucking in your gut or standing on one leg while performing a standing shoulder press. If you incorporate balance and stability training in your daily activities, you will need to intensely train your core only minimally.

Start being mindful of your core when you are performing activities, such as drawing your belly button in toward the small of your back. You'll look like you're sucking in your gut, but that action alone engages your core and therefore strengthens it. And you can do this small exercise while driving to work, sitting in your office, standing in line, or lying down reading a book. Sometimes I wear a form-fitting top to keep me mindful to "suck it in" throughout the day! So, attempt to hold your core for 3 or 4 minutes at a time, until you build your strength and the action becomes instinctive. Being mindful of your core will burn extra calories and improve your posture, but it needs to be supported with intense core training exercises, like planks, supermans, and bicycles.

MY TOP CORE TIPS

Here are some tips that will help improve your posture, burn fat, strengthen your core, and develop a toned midsection. Combined with a healthy diet and exercise plan, you can start seeing results within three weeks. (For illustrations of these moves, see pages 109 and 111.)

1. Engage your core for 3 minutes three times a day. Here is an exercise to remind yourself to engage your core. Inhale and imagine drawing in your belly button toward the small of your back. Exhale and watch your belly tighten. Do this small exercise while sitting in your office chair, standing in line at the grocery store, or walking to the mailbox. Tighten your belly and imagine your core muscles hardening. That's engagement.

2. Perform three exercises that focus on your transverse abdominals (TVA) three times a week. Your TVA are the deepest core muscles in your body. You can't see them but you will always feel them the next day after a deep core workout. The very best exercise for the TVA are variations of the plank, like pikes and side planks.

3. Perform 30 repetitions with 30-second breaks. Core muscles are used all the time, so focus on total engagement for a sustained period of time. Breaks should last only 30 seconds.

4. Train your lower back twice a week. Supermans, dead lifts, and back extensions are great exercises to strengthen the lower back. Perform three sets of 15 to 20 repetitions twice a week. If you commit to a lower back program, your abdominal area will notice a huge difference.

PRACTICE BREATHING PROPERLY

You should always exhale during the "hard" phase. For example, when you are performing a toe touch or bicycle crunch (see page 94), you exhale when you crunch. When you are performing an active superman (see page 97), you exhale when you raise your arms and legs.

Core Truth #3: Core work must engage the lower back and abdominal muscles.

Very often we are looking at only what we see in the mirror, which is usually our front. It's not an accident that most people fail to train their back, hamstrings, and calves. You just don't see them as much! You have to remember that our bodies are an entire unit made up of different parts. Our thighs, for example, can flex and extend because both the hamstrings (the back of the leg) and the quadriceps (the front of the leg) are performing the action. This is the same concept for the abdominals. To strengthen one side, you must equally engage the other side.

One of the best exercises to activate your back is the *superman* (see page 264). You lie on your stomach and raise your arms and legs at the same time. If you want to make it more challenging, try incorporating some movement by raising your legs and arms up and down simultaneously for 15 to 20 repetitions. This lower-back exercise elongates and stretches the front of your body and assists in the overall development of your abdominal muscles.

Core Truth #4: The core's most often the LAST place you will see develop.

Many people have heard the phrase "abs are made in the kitchen." It's true to the extent that it requires a disciplined diet to burn the last 10 pounds of fat sticking to your body. Your body doesn't know you want to look sexy in a swimsuit or fit into your high school jeans. It just wants to survive, and so it stores extra energy in the form of fat as a safety precaution. That's why losing the last 10 pounds to uncover your abdominal muscles is so difficult—it goes against your body's natural instinct for self-preservation. Seeing your abdominal muscles pop will require you to be at a lower body fat percentage, which can be attained only by eating a very healthy diet and committing to an intense exercise routine that will speed up your metabolism.

Let's Talk About Strength

Strength training is all about control. It's about challenging your body with the right amount of opposition, without straining yourself. It's about becoming stronger because your core is stronger. It's about increasing your flexibility, your bone strength, and your metabolism.

There are two types of exercise: aerobic and anaerobic. *Aerobic exercise* uses oxygen, and therefore glycogen and fat storage, to meet the physical demands of your body. You engage in aerobic exercise when you perform long durations of light to moderate cardio activities. *Anaerobic exercise,* also known as *strength training,* doesn't use oxygen for energy. Instead, it depends primarily on your glycogen storage (food) to provide quick energy to train at maximum exertion. You cannot sustain anaerobic exercise for a long period of time, which is why you need to rest between strength sets. Aerobic and anaerobic training are equally important when designing your fitness program.

You need to create a strength-training program that works for you. I don't like promoting the latest fad workout DVD or exercise class, because a workout plan should fit your own strengths and weaknesses. If you can lift heavy objects and perform intense exercise without mental or muscular fatigue, you are strong in that area. If you notice imbalances in your posture, weakness in your muscles, tightness in your tendons, or irregular pain in a static position, then these are areas you need to improve.

There is a lot of information to decipher on the Internet, especially some advice that is contradictory. As a general rule, I like to keep things simple. So here are some fundamentals to remember:

1. MORE MUSCLE INCREASES YOUR METABOLISM. Unlike fat tissue, muscle is an active tissue that requires more nutrients to sustain itself. Having more muscle speeds up your metabolism, which allows you to eat more (who wouldn't love that?). For example, see the following graph:

ORGAN OR TISSUE	DAILY METABOLIC RATE
Adipose (fat)	2 calories per pound
Muscle	6 calories per pound
Liver	91 calories per pound
Brain	109 calories per pound
Heart	200 calories per pound
Kidneys	200 calories per pound

2. 1 POUND OF MUSCLE IS SMALLER THAN 1 POUND OF FAT. Muscle is more compact than fat and so, pound for pound, is nearly three times smaller than an equal amount of fat. This is important to remember when you're weighing yourself and not seeing the scale budge while your measurements are dropping. Use other measurements for success and don't be a slave to the scale.

3. WOMEN HAVE A HARDER TIME BUILDING MUSCLE THAN MEN. Women who say they are afraid of looking like a bodybuilder don't understand how a woman's body works. Women don't have the same amount of testosterone that men have to build incredibly large muscles. If you want to "tone up," then strength training, or building muscle, is key. If you want to look lean, then decrease the fat on top of the muscle by following a balanced cardio and strength routine. In short, you can't be lean if you have no muscle. Do you see the problem here? You need to weight-train or you can't look toned.

4. THERE ARE THREE WAYS TO CONTRACT YOUR MUSCLES.

There are three ways to contract, and therefore challenge, your muscles: concentric, eccentric, and isometric movement. The *concentric* concentrates on shortening the muscle, which is the phase most lifters focus on. The *eccentric* decelerates the muscle. The *isometric* is static, when the muscle is held in a challenging position. For example, when you raise your body from a squat, you are performing a concentric motion; when you lower your body into a squat, you are performing an eccentric motion; and when you hold your body in a challenging squat, you are performing an isometric motion.

BUILDING MUSCLE

When designing a strength program, you start with the basic body-weight exercises like push-ups, squats, and sit-ups; and you adjust the degree of difficulty as you become stronger. In my earliest training years I performed a whole-body circuit two or three times a week. When my body adjusted to that challenge, I focused on pushing exercises one day (chest/shoulders/triceps) and pulling exercises the next day (back and biceps). As my body continued to adapt, I switched to one major body part a day (this is when I also had more time) or I incorporated other tools to make the exercises more challenging.

You will need to identify which stage you are currently in so as to select a safe but challenging strength-training routine. As you get stronger, you will find that you can make your body work harder by increasing the resistance your body is dealing with. As you become more confident in your workouts, think about challenging yourself by stepping up your resistance using the following:

Stage One: Body Weight

You don't need special equipment to challenge your body. Most often, all you need is your own body weight. Think push-ups, pull-ups, squats, lunges, dips, and sit-ups (see the Appendix). These major strength exercises don't require an exercise machine or a gym membership. Many popular home workout DVDs focus on plyometric body-weight exercises. All you need, though, is good form, an indelible motivation, and a goal.

MACHINES

While I'm not a big fan of machines, because it's easy to forget to engage the core when using them, I did start my fitness life using machines because they taught me the motion of the muscles. At most gyms you will find a circuit of machines lined up next to one another that perform specific actions. Read the directions, look at the visual, adjust the equipment (because it's not made for everyone's body type), and use a weight that is challenging.

Stage Two: Cables

Cables are freestanding and require you to use more of your core and central nervous system. Free-motion machines and Bowflexes have this cable component. Besides the concentric motion, exercises on these machines specifically challenge the eccentric motion of your body because the cables require you to control your decelerated movement.

Stage Three: Free Weights

Free weights in the form of barbells, dumbbells, or kettlebells engage your entire body, including your central nervous system, because they require you to control the weight, to balance your body, and to engage your core. This is the easiest and most affordable strength equipment to incorporate into a home routine as long as the weights are heavy enough to produce good tension.

Stage Four: Any Weight Plus Instability

Remember, strength training is all about control. The less controlled your environment is, the more your body will gain through the adversity. Start creating more imbalances by performing a shoulder press on one leg or a chest press while lying on a stability ball. Stand on a box while performing alternating dumbbell bicep curls or a lunge with your back foot raised. The more unstable you are, the more you're forced to engage.

SOME POPULAR STRENGTH WORKOUTS

1. *TRX.* TRX is a popular suspension training workout that has a variety of exercises for the entire body. It focuses on moving your body in multiple planes of motion while engaging your core and challenging your muscles simultaneously.

2. *CrossFit.* CrossFit and the WOD (workout of the day) focuses on overall conditioning, Olympic weight lifting, kettlebells, flipping tires, climbing ropes, and other challenging conditioning exercises that are more anaerobic in nature.

3. *Pilates.* Pilates can be performed on a mat or a reformer. It focuses on engaging your core while performing small repetitive movements that increase muscle endurance.

4. *Yoga.* Yoga works the entire body and focuses on core, flexibility, overall strength, and balance. You work through several isometric poses to strengthen your body and engage your mind.

WALKING ONTO THE WEIGHT ROOM FLOOR

It's intimidating to walk onto the weight room floor with men grunting, iron clinking, and everyone focusing on his or her toned physique in the mirrors. While difficult, you must do what scares you. I was scared at first—everyone is at one point! The best way to overcome this fear is to educate yourself and then just do it. Start getting comfortable with the movement of your muscles by using the

Here are some tips to keep in mind before you start to train. I often say it's hard to break bad habits, so instead create new ones the right way.

THINGS TO KEEP IN MIND BEFORE YOU TRAIN!

1. *Use a challenging weight.* On a scale of 1 to 10 (10 being the heaviest), you should be working at a level 7 or 8 and be very fatigued (level 9) by the last couple of reps. To build muscle, there must be enough resistance to create strength. Everyone's level will be different, but don't be afraid to push yourself a little bit out of your comfort zone!

2. *Alter your repetitions in accordance to your physical goals.* Focus on shorter repetitions between 8 and 12 for building muscle and 12 and 18 for maintaining muscle.

3. *Time your rest periods.* They should last only around 30 to 45 seconds between sets. If you are concentrating on building muscle, you should rest 2 to 3 minutes to ensure you are fully recovered from your last set.

4. *Maintain good posture by finding your 90-degree angle.* A 90-degree angle comes naturally in your movement, so seek it. Keep a 90-degree angle as you squat, lunge, push-up, and press—you will see it everywhere.

5. *Concentrate on your breathing.* Exhale through the hard/concentric phase of your movement and inhale during the easy/eccentric phase. For example, if you are performing a squat, you must exhale as your body rises

from a squatted position to an upright standing position. When you exhale, you are engaging your core, which assists in your overall power during the exercise.

6. *Practice full extension.* Execute a complete range of motion when performing any exercise. When performing a bicep curl, for example, you want to raise the weight and flex to a point where you see your bicep muscle peak. As soon as it peaks, slowly lower your forearm until your arm is almost fully extended.

7. *Don't lock your joints.* When you lock out, you not only rest your muscle during an exercise but also apply pressure to your joints, which eventually causes strain and possible injury.

8. *Start with good posture.* You should have your chest up, shoulders back, core tight, lower back slightly arched, hips squared, and feet forward. If you start with good posture, you will move and end (you hope) with good posture!

9. *Play with your angles.* Target different areas of the muscle. By shifting your angle a small degree, you can target a different area of your muscle.

10. *If you feel sharp or throbbing pain (bad pain), STOP!* Injuries are not only a pain in the butt, but they will slow your progress, so the best thing to do is avoid them by using good form, engaging your core, and being mindful. If you feel any pain, immediately stop and allow your body to recover before engaging in the activity again.

machines, observe the exercises performed by other people, and ask questions! Everyone at the gym is there for the same reason, so don't be shy. Get comfortable with being uncomfortable.

Using the illustrated list of exercises in the Appendix, pick two or three body parts and perform two or three exercises for each one. Depending on your goal, you can either choose 12 to 15 repetitions for weight loss or 8 to 12 repetitions for strength. You can divide your strength training into days you train just your upper body, then your lower body the following day. If you want to change it up, you can get more technical and perform all pulling exercises like rows, flies, and curls on one day and pushing exercises like presses, squats, and extensions on the next day. Some people pick one body part a day or a full body workout a few times a week. You need to experiment and find what's best for you.

For those who don't have a gym membership, invest in some weights or resistance bands at home so you can follow the same exercises utilizing your home equipment, or make your own weights—think discarded milk gallons filled with sand! I've used my own children as weights (that was fun) and water bottles for hand weights!

Let's Talk About Cardio

If you want to lose weight, you can't skrimp on cardio. Cardiovascular exercise strengthens your heart, increases your metabolism, promotes happy hormones, and prevents heart disease. As long as your heart is pumping, your blood is flowing and your body is moving, you are engaging in life-extending activity. Many people falsely believe the only way to exercise is by running, taking a Zumba class, using an elliptical, or performing a workout DVD.

No.

Cardio is whatever challenges your body in its target heart rate (THR) which is 220 minus your age multiplied by 55 to 85 percent of your maximum heart rate. For example, as I write this I am 33 years old. My maximum heart rate is 187 bpm (beats per minute) and my target heart rate is 102 to 158 beats per minute.

You can jog in place, perform continuous squats, or dance at your THR for 20 minutes, and that's considered cardio! What's most important is that you focus, stay engaged, and calculate your heart rate every few minutes to ensure you are training hard enough.

There are so many ways to get your cardio in. I sometimes perform jumping jacks, jump rope, or do step-ups at the park while I watch my children play. While waiting between flights at the airport I have walked up and down flights of stairs. In a hotel room without any access to a gym, I have found some workout videos on YouTube. You can always find a way to incorporate cardio exercise if you're willing to get a little creative and not take no for an answer!

Have you ever seen someone talk on the phone, read a novel, or watch TV while he or she is on a treadmill? This isn't even breathing hard! *Don't be that person.* The No More Excuses journey is about efficiency, and you don't want to waste your time training if you're not training hard enough. You should be working up a sweat and feeling a little winded, but still be able to talk.

You can monitor your heart rate by using the heart rate sensor on most cardio equipment. You can also wear a heart rate monitor or be old school (like me) and take your pulse on the side of your neck or along the veins of your wrist. Count the beats there for 15 seconds and multiply by 4. That magic number is how many times your heart beats per minute.

Cardio exercise can be simple, fun, accessible, and challenging. And it doesn't have to be boring! Anything that gets your heart rate up for an extended period of time is considered cardio. In general, your exercise program should reflect both your strengths and your weaknesses. Throughout my training week I perform something physically difficult like running (hard) and taking dance class (easy). I mix up these forms of cardio to prevent boredom and to sustain my motivation. Nontraditional cardio activities include hiking, swimming, skating, climbing, and biking. As long as your heart is engaged and your body and mind are challenged, you are having a good workout.

The calories you burn per minute depend on your age, amount of muscle, metabolism, intensity, and weight. The more muscle and overall weight you have, the more calories you will burn performing aerobic activity. Here are some great cardio options:

CLASSES
Dancing
Kickboxing
Martial arts
Spinning
Step
Swimming
Zumba

CARDIO MACHINES
Arc trainer
Elliptical
Rower
Stairmaster
Stationary bike
Treadmill
Upright bike
VersaTREK

BODY-WEIGHT ACTIVITIES
Jumping rope
Lunges
Squats
Swings

RECREATIONAL ACTIVITIES
Biking
Canoeing
Hiking
Roller-skating
Surfing

One thing a lot of people don't realize is that training for a race is not the best way to lose weight. A lot of people make it a goal to run a 5K, 10K, or half-marathon to lose weight, but while that is a great fitness goal, it may not be the best weight-loss goal. Your heart, body, and spirit will definitely get stronger in the process, but if you want to lose weight, then watch your caloric intake. You may lose weight in the process of running more, but remember that running more might mean eating more. Eating more means you aren't leaving the caloric deficit that is needed for weight loss.

CARDIO IS PERFORMED AFTER STRENGTH TRAINING

Cardio should be performed after your warm-up and strength training. This is because you want your body to utilize your glycogen storage (carbohydrates found in your muscle) to pull, press, and push weights. Since strength training is the more intense part of your routine, you want to make sure most of your stored energy is expelled during that period. I make it a general rule to train no longer than 90 minutes at a time, and I recommend you do the same, as your body will require fuel. If you don't properly feed yourself, your performance suffers, your results decline, and your efforts are wasted.

Making efficient effort is the crux of the No More Excuses program. Success is not how often you do something; it's how well you do it. Here are some handy tips for getting the most from your cardio workout.

1. Short intense intervals are the best type of cardio.

As a busy mom, I was relieved to read that the overwhelming number of studies shows that shorter cardio durations incorporating interval training burn more calories after training than do longer low-intensity cardio activities. That is, slow and steady sometimes wins the race, but in this case fast and challenging gets the reward. I usually start by warming up for 5 to 10 minutes, then change my intensity every 30 to 45 seconds, whereby my heart is challenged for a short duration and then recovers for an amount of equal time. I perform intervals for a minimum of 20 minutes.

2. For long-term results, you can't just focus on cardio training.

Raise your hand if you are a cardio queen or king! Raise both hands if you love taking group exercise classes and hardly ever step onto the weight room floor. While cardio is definitely beneficial for your lungs and heart, to create and sustain results, you need to balance strength and cardio training. I promise you, you will notice that people who stopped taking cardio classes and got comfortable with the free weights outside the classroom are the ones who finally started seeing results.

Perform a minimum of 20 minutes for three or four days a week. When you hit a plateau, increase your duration, change your intensity, or switch your exercise.

CARDIO TRAINING TIPS!

1. *Change your workout every three weeks.* If you are used to running a 12-minute mile, try running at an 11-minute pace or increase your incline. There is no change without challenge.

2. *Listen to upbeat music.* Studies have shown that listening to music stimulates the motor area of your brain, which promotes greater physical intensity.

3. *Experiment with different group exercise classes.* When you are unmotivated, being with others gets your blood pumping. It also adds a degree of fun to your workout.

4. *Purchase easy and inexpensive home equipment.* Include a jump rope or workout DVD. The convenience will give you little excuse for not fitting in your 20-minute workout.

5. *Get outside.* The best kind of workout is in open terrain, where you breathe fresh air and are one with nature. Being outside creates a less stable environment as well, which stimulates your central nervous system and challenges your body and mind. Running, jogging, hiking, swimming, and biking are all great activities to perform outdoors.

Let's Stretch!

Flexibility training is often overlooked, but it is incredibly important. We take advantage of our abilities to bend, reach, grab, and turn. However, as you get older, your body's agility and elasticity change. While the jury is out on whether great flexibility prevents injuries, I will say that the more flexible you are, the more joint mobility you have. The greater your body's range of motion, the smaller your risk of straining a muscle. Certain muscles start getting tight, specific movements become shorter, and your body's ability to move freely grows limited. Stretching relieves muscle soreness, opens up circulation, and reduces stress.

Stretching should be performed after you have warmed up for 5 to 10 minutes or after your entire workout. To get a really good stretch, you should get the blood circulating and your muscles warmed.

> When performing a stretch, follow proper form and hold the stretch for at least 12 to 15 seconds. Don't hold your breath. Make sure you are slowly inhaling and exhaling, especially as you reach farther to deepen your stretch.

Seeking balance in your strength, cardio, and flexibility routines is tough. For many people, stretching is definitely the challenging part—after all, when you have completed an exhausting workout, the last thing you want to do is spend additional minutes stretching. Nevertheless, here are some speedy thoughts to make you a better stretcher:

1. Stretching can be done any time of the day.

You don't need to be in a gym, wearing athletic shoes and a sports bra, to stretch. You can stretch in your office chair, while watching television, or between loads of laundry. While I recommend warming up to promote blood circulation before deep stretching sessions, smaller yet still beneficial stretching sessions can be performed anywhere.

2. Tight muscles, especially with a muscle imbalance, need the most stretching.

Most often you can match people's occupations with the kind of muscle soreness they may be experiencing. Most people who sit all day have tight chest and neck muscles. Most nurses and caregivers have lower back tension. Many runners experience tight hip flexors. Whatever conditions you impose on your body daily will be compensated for by muscle imbalances and eventually injury. Whenever I am conscious of my goals, I sit up straight in my chair while writing and stretch my neck and chest. I also take that opportunity to fix my posture. I do this while at stoplights or waiting in line at the grocery store, as well.

3. Practice yoga.

When you perform several sun salutations, you are challenging your body in various positions and holding it for a couple minutes. This not only strengthens your core and challenges your central nervous system, but it also focuses your breathing, loosens your muscles, and strengthens your body.

So how do you stretch? There are several types of stretching, but specifically four that you will engage in: ballistic, dynamic, self-myofascial release, and static.

Ballistic stretching is moving with momentum and stretching the muscle to its maximum. Imagine a small "bouncing" movement while performing a stretch—that's ballistic! An example of a ballistic stretch is when you sit in a straddle position and reach to one toe while bouncing back and forth to reach farther.

Dynamic stretching is a controlled action in which you slowly perform the movement. It prepares you for action and focuses on a full range of motion. An example of a dynamic stretch is when you perform unweighted squats before performing weighted squats.

Self-myofascial release, or SMR, stretching is becoming more commonly known these days. You apply pressure to the muscle via a foam roller while the muscle is relaxed. An example of an SMR stretch is sitting down on the ground with a foam roller beneath your tight hamstrings while your legs are positioned in a pike position.

Static stretching is the most common, what we generally learn in gym classes. You get into a stretch position and slowly stretch until you feel tension. You hold the position for several seconds, then release. An example of a static stretch is placing your arm behind your neck and dropping your forearm down while applying some tension with your other arm for a good triceps stretch.

I have used every form of stretching during and after my workouts depending on what feels best for my body. For deeper pain, I use SMR stretching by foam-rolling my upper back, glutes, or hamstrings. When I'm going to perform plyometrics, I use ballistic stretching to prepare my body for movement. When I'm warming up for a kickboxing class, I use dynamic stretching to loosen my legs. After an intense workout, I usually perform static stretches, especially along my trunk and legs.

Check out the stretching motions shown in the Appendix; these are my favorite stretches—a great way to reward yourself after a workout!

Put It All Together

On pages 94–127 you will find a variety of sample workouts, but you should also feel free to design your own. The guidelines presented in this chapter will help you develop your personal workout routine. I don't believe there is any single technique that will transform your body the most; a balanced program complete with a few training lessons is essential for becoming your strongest, fittest self. To get the most out of your exercise plan, devote three days to strength training and three days to performing cardio (they can be on the same day). You will then also perform flexibility training for 5 to 10 minutes at the end of each workout.

1. ***Stay hydrated.*** Don't work out without a water bottle. You are losing a lot of water while you exercise, so between sets make sure you're hydrating your body, allowing the water to replenish your cells. Try also squeezing some lemon into your water to add flavor, which will aid digestion and boost your immunity at the same time.

2. ***Focus on proper form.*** You should always be in control of your body when you work out, whether you're lifting, using a machine, or biking. If you are swinging your body, lacking control, and slouching during a strength exercise, then you are being counterproductive. Make sure your chest is high, shoulders are back, hips are squared, tummy is tight, and toes are forward. As you move your body through an exercise, maintain good posture; as soon as it starts to change, stop and identify your limited range of motion until you become stronger and more flexible.

3. ***Warm up for 5 to 10 minutes before strength training.*** Wake up your body and get your blood flowing. Warm up by walking at a fast pace, riding a bike, performing some step-ups, or using a jump rope. Not only will it stretch your limbs and joints, but it

will also awaken your mind and prepare you for a focused workout.

4. **Perform a minimum of 20 to 40 minutes of strength training three times a week.** Strength training is the fountain of youth for a lot of people. It molds your physique, makes your limbs strong, and keeps your metabolism churning. Building muscle can be completed by utilizing your own body weight, free weights, or machines at the gym.

5. **Perform intense cardio a minimum of 20 minutes at least three times a week.** Performing regular cardio not only builds a healthier heart but also burns your fat tissue. A healthy heart enables you to move blood through your veins and arteries with efficiency.

6. **Perform cardio on an empty stomach.** When you perform cardio you are burning either glycogen (food) or stored fat; when you do it on an empty stomach, you're going to start burning more stored fat faster! If you plan to perform morning cardio on an empty stomach, do so within the hour after you wake up. Otherwise, eat something, as your body has fasted for several hours while sleeping and needs food to function. If you decide to perform cardio later in the day, minimize your food intake a couple hours before your workout to ensure you are burning stored fat (and not what you just ate).

7. **Eat a carbohydrate within the hour before strength training.** When you are strength training, your body needs energy to lift, pull, and push. Carbohydrates are eaten for energy, so give your body an extra boost before you work out. I typically eat a piece of fruit or some oatmeal before a workout, but I ensure that my intake isn't too heavy, as a full stomach creates bloating, cramps, and indigestion.

8. **Eat protein and carbohydrates within an hour after training.** Carbohydrates are required to refuel your glycogen storage,

your body's main fuel, which is found in your muscles. Pairing your carbohydrates with a protein source will control your insulin levels and slow your digestion. Consuming both will refuel your glycogen stores and rebuild your muscle breakdown that occurred during your workout.

9. **_Stretch after you work out._** Stretching will prevent you from feeling sore after a workout; it also aids in the recovery process. It is an opportunity to relax, focus on your breathing, and get into a Zen zone before moving forward with your day.

10. **_Don't skimp on rest days._** Rest is very important for your body to heal and rejuvenate. Overtraining is a real danger, as you can feel depressed and irritable from chronic soreness and fatigue. If you are a beginner, try resting every other day. As you become more advanced, rest every third day. When you are intermediate, rest every fifth or sixth day. If you are sore, do not train the sore muscles. Lie in a bath of Epsom salt, stretch your tight muscles, and perform some light cardio to get your blood flowing.

SEVEN SAMPLE HOME WORKOUTS

When you are new to exercise you must slowly build your strength and endurance. Do not rush into any fitness activity too quickly, and make sure you always get your doctor's consent. You will train anywhere between three and six days per week. After three weeks your body will start adjusting to your program, so I have offered progressive workouts to change things up. Most of the exercises are demonstrated using proper form in the Appendix. Throughout my years training, I have cycled through these various workout programs and have changed them up by performing different exercises, adding supersets, increasing weights, altering reps/sets, or extending my workout duration (right now I'm at the Circuit Training phase again!).

On cardio days perform 20 to 45 minutes of cardio. If you lack time (as I often do), just perform 20 minutes but make sure you incorporate high-intensity interval training. At the end of each workout, include a small stretching routine that focuses on muscles worked and corrective postural stretches.

Each strength-training workout option is designed to challenge you and switch up your overall routine. Every three weeks, you can either change your intensity level, exercises, workout duration, strength routine, or training structure.

There are three common training structures. Each training structure is designed to challenge the muscle depending on an individual's goals and experience level. Choose your strength routine, cardio exercise, and training structure, and get ready to work hard. Here are various workouts to keep your body guessing every 3 weeks for the next 12 weeks.

Training Structures

STRAIGHT SETS

Keep the weight constant through your entire exercise. This is great for beginners to learn form and build muscular endurance.

SET	WEIGHT	REPS
1	10 pounds	10
2	10 pounds	10
3	10 pounds	10

PYRAMID SETS

This is the most conventional type of training, in which you decrease your repetitions as your weight increases. This method focuses on overloading and exhausting the muscle so it creates fatigue.

SET	WEIGHT	REPS
1	10 pounds	12
2	15 pounds	10
3	20 pounds	8

REVERSE PYRAMID SETS

Properly warm up before tackling the hardest weight first. This training utilizes your energy to build muscle by emphasizing the first sets versus the last.

SET	WEIGHT	REPS
1	20 pounds	8
2	10 pounds	10
3	8 pounds	12

Push exercises engage the chest, shoulders, triceps, quadriceps, calves, and glutes; pull exercises engage the back, biceps, and hamstrings.

Workout Chart Abbreviations

BW: Body weight

DB: Dumbbells

MB: Medicine ball

RB: Resistance band

SB: Stability ball

ACTIVE REST: Recreational activity like hiking, swimming, playing tennis, etc.

DROP SET: Performing one exercise until failure and completing an additional set with lower weight without rest.

SUPER SET: Performing two exercises back-to-back without rest.

Whole-Body Circuit Training

The first stage when incorporating strength training into your workout is to begin with a whole-body circuit. If you are a beginner, start here. As your core gets stronger and your posture improves, you can begin tackling more progressive workouts. If you own fitness DVDs or enjoy attending group classes, you can incorporate these workouts as part of your circuit training on Monday, Wednesday, and Friday. If you exercise at home and have some equipment, here are a couple workouts to include for the first three weeks of your program.

HOME WORKOUT 1

SUNDAY: Rest

MON/WED/FRI: 20 to 45 Minutes of Cardio
Perform 3 sets of each exercise below, using the training structure you've chosen from page 92.

ARMS
BW Push-up

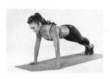

Squatting
RB Back Row

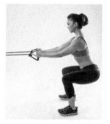

DB Shoulder
Press

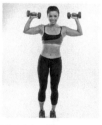

Standing
RB Alternating
Bicep Curl

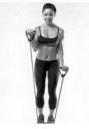

DB Tricep
Extension

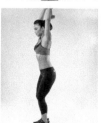

LEGS
BW Lunge

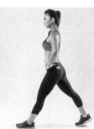

BW Plie Squat

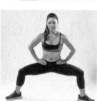

ABS
BW Toe Touch

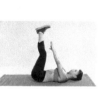

BW Bicycle
Crunch

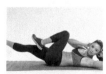

BW Plank

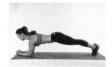

TUES/THU: Rest or 20 to 45 Minutes of Cardio

STRETCH EXERCISES

Child's Pose
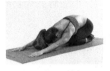

Lying Hamstrings
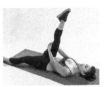

Cat
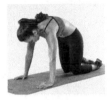

Lying Spinal Twist
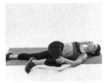

Cow
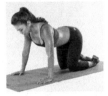

Lying Glutes

Hip Flexors
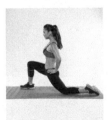

Seated Arm Circles

Lying Knees to Chest
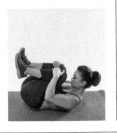

SATURDAY: Rest

HOME WORKOUT 2

SUNDAY: Rest

MON/WED/FRI: 20 to 45 Minutes of Cardio
Perform 3 sets of each exercise below, using the training structure you've chosen from page 92.

ARMS

Lying DB Chest Press

DB Bent-over Row

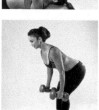

Squatted Alternating DB Shoulder Press

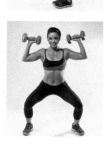

DB Bicep Curl with Lunge

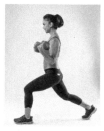

BW Chair Triceps Dip

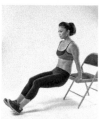

(continued on next page)

LEGS
BW Squat
Jump

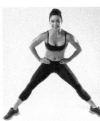

BACK
DB Dead Lift

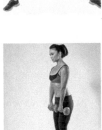

CORE
BW Toe Touch

BW Russian
Twist

BW Reverse
Crunch

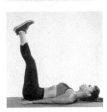

BW Superman

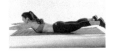

TUES/THU: Rest or 20 to 45 Minutes of Cardio

STRETCH EXERCISES

Neck

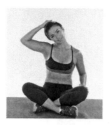

Chest

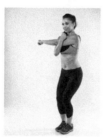

Shoulders

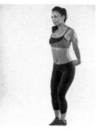

Triceps

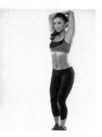

Legs

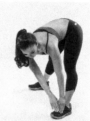

Standing
Glutes

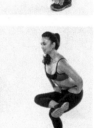

Standing
Quads

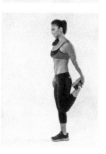

SATURDAY: Rest

Upper and Lower Split Training

This training involves focusing on specific muscles by dividing your body in to upper and lower halves. When you concentrate on several exercises dedicated to a specific region of the body, it creates muscular fatigue, atrophy, and eventually additional strength.

HOME WORKOUT 3

SUNDAY: Rest

MON/THU: 20 to 45 Minutes of Cardio

UPPER BODY

Perform 3 sets of each exercise below, using the training structure you've chosen from page 92.

BW Push-up

Lying DB Chest Fly

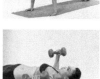

Kneeling RB Lat Pull-down

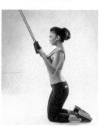

Squatting RB Back Row

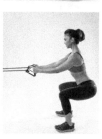

DB Shoulder Press

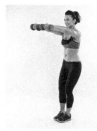

DB Front Raise

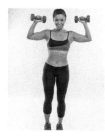

DB Side Raise

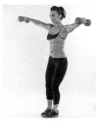

DB Reverse Fly

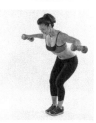

(continued on next page)

DB Bicep Curl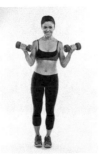

Shoulders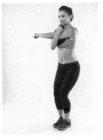

Standing
DB Tricep
Extension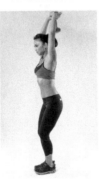

Triceps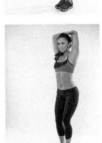

Neck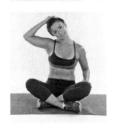

Stretch Exercises

Chest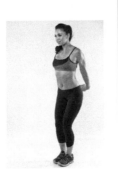

TUES/FRI: 20 to 45 Minutes of Cardio

LOWER BODY

Perform 3 sets of each exercise below, using the training structure you've chosen from page 92.

BW Lunge Jump

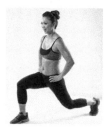

DB Calf Raise

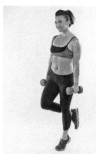

BW Side Lunge

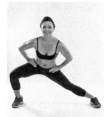

BW Step-up

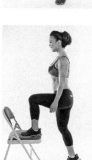

BW Star Jump

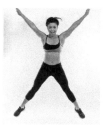

BW Glute Bridge

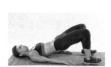

BW Plie Squat

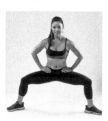

Stretch Exercises

Legs

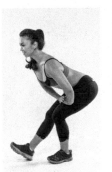

Standing
Quads

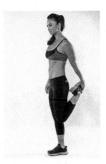

Hamstrings

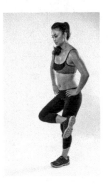

Standing
Glutes

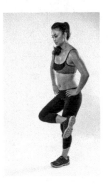

WEDNESDAY: 20 to 45 Minutes of Cardio

CORE WORK

Perform 3 sets of each exercise below, using the training structure you've chosen from page 92.

BW Plank
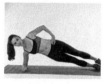

BW Bicycle Crunch
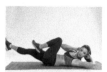

BW Side Plank
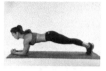

BW Reverse Crunch
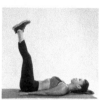

BW Superman
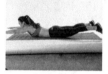

BW Toe Touch
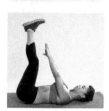

Push and Pull Split

As your body becomes more accustomed to training with weights, it will require you to keep it guessing. Adding a push and pull exercise split will force muscles with similar operational functions to fatigue from overwhelming stress.

HOME WORKOUT 4

SUNDAY: Rest

MON/THU: PUSH: Chest/Shoulders/Triceps/Quads and 20 to 45 Minutes of Cardio

Lying DB Chest Press
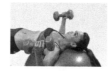

Kneeling RB Chest Press
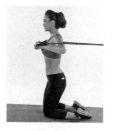

Squatted Alternating DB Shoulder Press
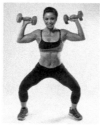

SUPERSET
DB Side Raise
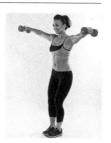

DB Front Raise
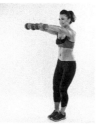

DB Standing Upright Row
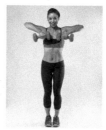

DB One-legged Overhead Tricep Extension
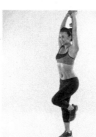

BW Chair Triceps Dip
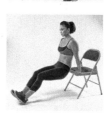

MB Squat Overhead Throw
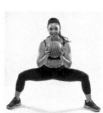

BW Squat Kick
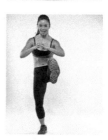

Stretch Exercises

Seated Arm
Circles

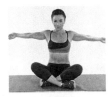

Lying Glutes

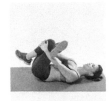

Neck

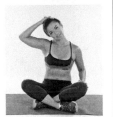

Inner Thighs

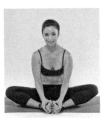

Lying
Hamstrings

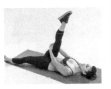

TUE/FRI: PULL: Back/Biceps/Hamstrings and 20 to 45 Minutes of Cardio

Stretch Exercises

Kneeling RB Lat Pull-down

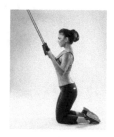

Chest

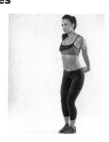

DB Bent-over Row

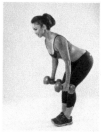

Neck

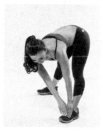

DB Standing Upright Row

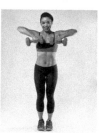

Legs

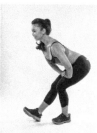

Standing RB Alternating Bicep Curl

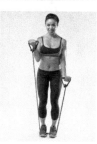

Hamstrings

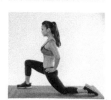

DB One-legged Dead Lift

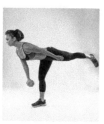

Hip Flexors

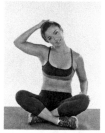

WEDNESDAY: Rest or 20 to 45 Minutes of Cardio

CORE WORK

Perform 3 sets of each exercise below, using the training structure you've chosen from page 92.

BW Plank

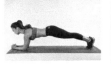

BW Bird Dog

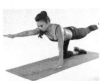

BW V-up

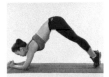

MB Curl-up

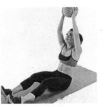

BW Side Plank

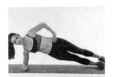

MB Russian Twist

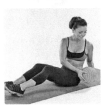

Individual Muscle Training

An intense option is to work a single muscle group and isolate it for the entire strength session. This will exhaust your muscle fibers and increase your strength.

HOME WORKOUT 5

SUNDAY: Rest

MONDAY: 20 to 45 Minutes of Cardio

CHEST
BW Push-up

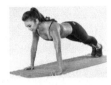

MB Push-up

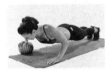

Lying DB
Pullover

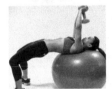

MB Chest Pass

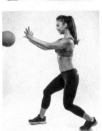

CORE
BW Plank

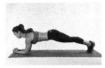

BW V-up

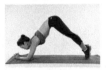

BW Side Plank

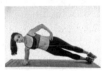

BW Superman

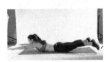

BW Russian
Twist

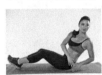

BW Reverse
Crunch

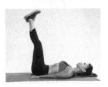

TUESDAY: Back and 20 to 45 Minutes of Cardio

Kneeling
RB Lat
Pull-down

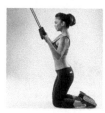

DB Bent-over
Row

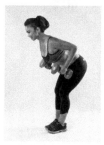

DB Lying Back
Pullover

DB One-
legged Dead
Lift

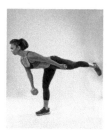

BW Superman

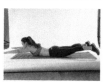

WEDNESDAY: Shoulders and 20 to 45 Minutes of Cardio

ARMS
DB Squatted
Alternating
Shoulder Press

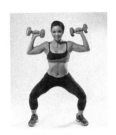

CORE
MB Curl-up

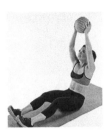

DB Standing
Upright Row

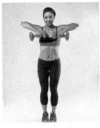

MB Russian
Twist

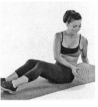

RB Standing
One-arm Front
Raise

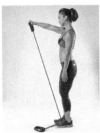

BW Flutter
Kick

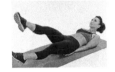

RB Standing
One-arm
Lateral Raise

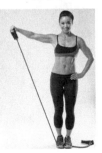

DB Reverse Fly

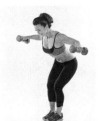

THURSDAY: 20 to 45 Minutes of Cardio

ARMS

DB Bicep Curl

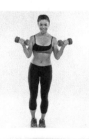

DB Single-legged Standing Bicep Curl

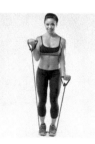

SUPERSET

RB Standing Alternating Bicep Curl

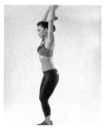

Standing DB Tricep Extension

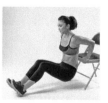

BW Chair Triceps Dip

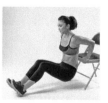

BW Close-grip Push-up

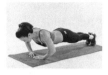

Stretch Exercises

Chest

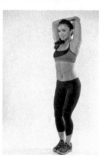

Triceps

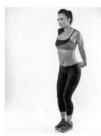

Neck

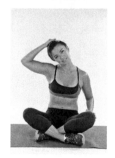

FRIDAY: 20 to 45 Minutes of Cardio

LEGS
BW Lunge

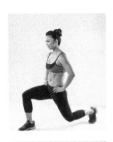

BW Lunge
Jump

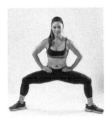

SUPERSET
BW Squat

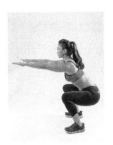

BW Plie Squat

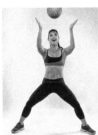

MB Squat
Overhead
Throw

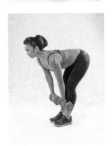

DB Dead Lift

SATURDAY: Rest or 20 to 45 Minutes of Cardio

Balance Training

If you find any of the training options too intense, try incorporating balance training. It will awaken your central nervous system while challenging your strength, endurance, and core.

HOME WORKOUT 6

SUNDAY: Rest

MONDAY: Strength/Balance/Plyometric Training and 20 to 45 Minutes of Cardio

MB Push-up

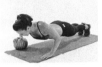

BW Jump Rope

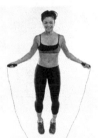

Kneeling RB Lat Pull-down

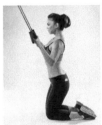

BW Jump Rope

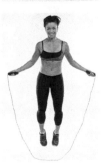

DB One-legged Shoulder Press

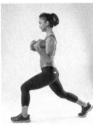

DB Bicep Curls with Lunge

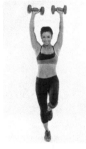

DB One-legged Overhead Tricep Extension

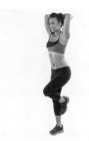

BW Lunge Jump

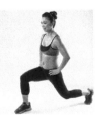

(continued on next page)

BW Reverse
Crunch

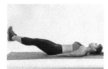

BW Squat
Jump

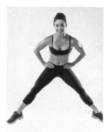

BW Bicycle
Crunch

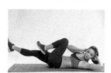

Stretch Exercises

Cat

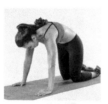

Cow

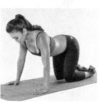

Child's Pose

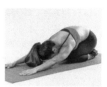

Hip Flexors

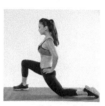

Seated Spinal
Twist

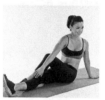

Neck

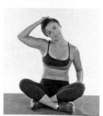

Seated Arm
Circles

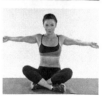

TUES/THURS: **Stretch Exercises**

Back

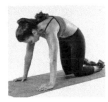

Lying Knee to Chest

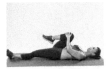

Lying Hamstrings

Lying Spinal Twist

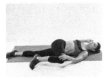

SMR IT Band

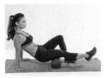

SMR Hamstrings

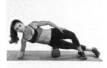

SMR Upper Back

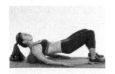

WEDNESDAY: Strength/Balance/Plyometric Training and 20 to 45 Minutes of Cardio

Lying DB Chest Fly

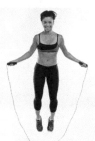

BW Jump Rope

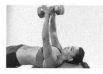

Squatting RB Back Row

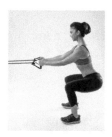

BW Jump Rope

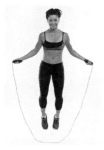

Squatted Alternating DB Shoulder Press

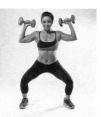

DB Bicep Curl with Lunge

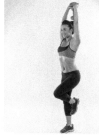

DB One-legged Overhead Tricep Extension

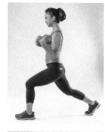

BW Lunge Jump

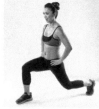

BW Reverse Crunch

BW Squat Jump

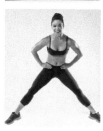

BW Bicycle Crunch

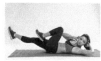

FRIDAY: Strength/Balance/Plyometric Training and 20 to 45 Minutes of Cardio

MB Chest Pass

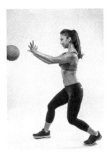

MB Push-up

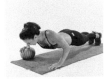

LEGS

MB Squat Overhead Throw

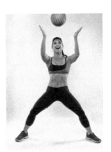

BW Star Jump

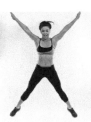

DB One-legged Dead Lift

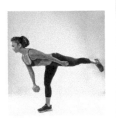

ABS

MB Russian Twist

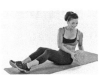

BW Bicycle Crunch

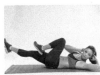

BW Flutter Kick

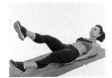

DB Bent-over Row

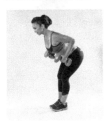

BW Step-up

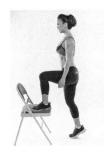

Cardio Interval Training

Incorporating intense intervals during a cardio routine can wake up your metabolism and increase your body's burn rate after it has finished training.

HOME WORKOUT 7

....

SUNDAY: Rest

MONDAY: 30-minute High-Intensity Cardio Training

3 SETS OF 1 MINUTE EACH, WITH 1-MINUTE REST BETWEEN SETS

BW Butt Kick
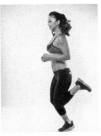

BW High Knee
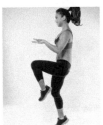

BW Star Jump
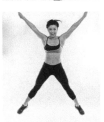

BW Lunge Jump
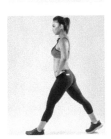

BW Squat
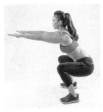

BW Plie Squat
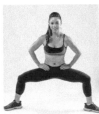

BW Jump Rope
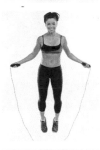

BW Plank
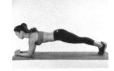

BW Step-up
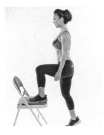

TUES/THUR: Low-Impact Cardio and Stretch

Lying Knees to Chest

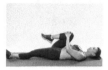

Lying Glutes

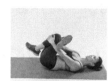

Back

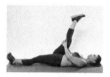

Inner Thighs

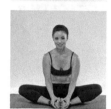

Lying Hamstrings

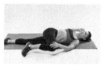

Neck

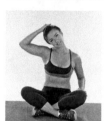

Lying Spinal Twist

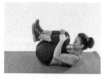

Seated Arm Circles

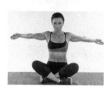

WEDNESDAY: 30-minute High-Intensity Cardio Training

3 SETS OF 1 MINUTE EACH, WITH 1-MINUTE REST BETWEEN SETS

BW Jump Rope

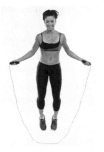

BW Curtsy
Lunge

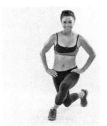

BW High Knee

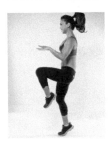

BW Butt Kick

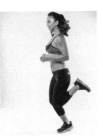

BW Star Jump

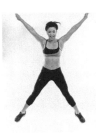

BW Mountain
Climber

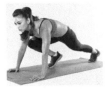

BW Squat

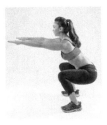

BW Push-up

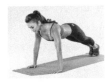

BW Bicycle
Crunch

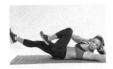

FRIDAY: 30-minute High-Intensity Cardio Training

3 SETS OF 1 MINUTE EACH, WITH 1-MINUTE REST BETWEEN SETS

BW Squat Kick

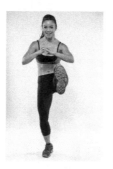

BW Frog Jump

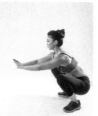

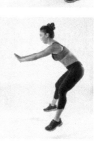

BW Step-up

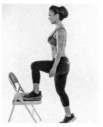

Jog in Place

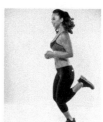

BW Push-up

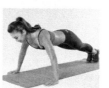

BW Squat
Jump

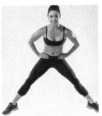

BW Side Lunge

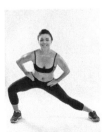

BW Squat

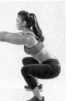

BW Mountain
Climber

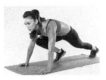

SATURDAY: Rest

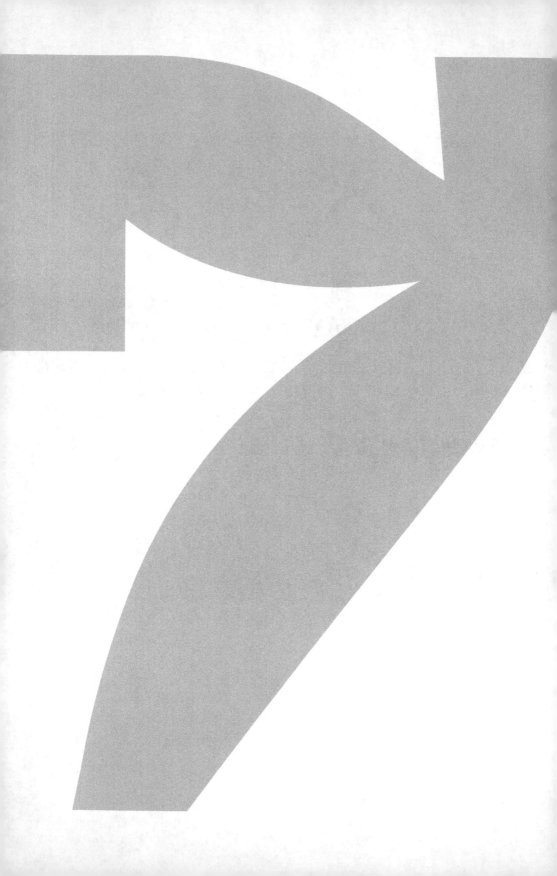

THE 80 PERCENT OF YOUR EFFORT

Your nutrition component is 80 percent of your results while your fitness is 20 percent. Food is the fuel that operates your body. Your body is set up to think, sleep, exercise, and move, and it needs food to do all that. Most of all, food is at the heart of every family event, holiday celebration, and special occasion. Food is an integral part of our lives, yet that single factor may be holding you back from reaching your best body. There are many quick fixes, detoxes, and extreme diets marketed today, but the only thing that works is an eating plan you can stick to in the long run. If your food intake isn't realistic, flexible, and achievable, then you haven't got the good eating routine you need for success and you will eventually fall short of meeting your goals.

I remember years ago watching Oprah Winfrey and seeing her guest, professional organizer Peter Walsh, say that we use 20 percent of our clothes 80 percent of the time. Wow! I thought about my favorite pair of jeans, workout pants, and tops and I had to agree. It was a big revelation for me and I began applying that formula to my health and fitness philosophy. My 80:20 outlook on exercise and diet coincides with the economic percentage known as the Pareto Principle, coined by Vilfredo Pareto in 1897, when he observed the pattern of distribution between wealth and income. He saw his society naturally divided into the "vital few," the 20 percent who had money and influence over the bottom 80 percent, who lacked resources. This relationship can be seen in many professional, personal, and physical settings.

In the past I thought I could outrun a bad diet. I would often treat myself to a sweet dessert after a hard workout! I thought that diet and exercise were equal, a perfect 50:50 in value and results. But after many failed diet attempts and more weight gain, I realized that diet is far more important than I originally thought. Even eating something seemingly healthy, like my favorite Subway sandwich with baked chips and a large raspberry ice tea, was more calories than I burned on my 3-mile run. If you are working out weekly and still drinking fancy coffee drinks, snacking on evening ice cream, and skipping breakfast, then you will see minimal results. Eighty percent of your weight-loss success will stem from your nutritional input, and the last 20 percent is from your exercise output.

The 80:20 principle doesn't mean you have to be perfect. As a past perfectionist who has struggled with her weight, I constantly felt like a failure when I splurged on my favorite foods several times a week while watching TV, enjoying happy hours, and attending family events. Indulging unexpectedly several times a week felt like a never-ending "starting line," where I would start anew every Monday, hoping to be perfect on my diet and exercise plan, only to finish the week in last place.

When I began incorporating the 80:20 principle into my life, though, I became more forgiving of my small setbacks—in fact, my setbacks began to be part of the plan! I began succeeding by eating healthy 80 percent of the time and allowing splurges 20 percent of the time. This new way of thinking allowed me to eat healthy throughout the week and to enjoy small planned treats during a weekday lunch or weekend event. Most of my friends and family were surprised I was losing weight while indulging at parties, not realizing that the majority of the time—when they rarely saw me—I was eating balanced, nutritious, and healthy meals.

The No More Excuses diet is a long-term healthy lifestyle. It's about striving to become a better person. But it includes failing—yes, failing! The idea is that you conduct S.P.E.E.D. trials in your fitness and nutritional goals and see what works. Then, you set your nutritional goals, plan your meals, envision your success, execute your plan, and deliver the results. Did you eat enough? Did you snack too much? If you want to succeed, you need to be forgiving of your occasional setbacks and flexible with your goals—and even your timeline. I know this from experimenting with nearly every diet that exists, and I finally found what works. I completed my S.P.E.E.D. strategy and I revised it weekly. There are a lot of dieting tactics out there, and all of them can become confusing very fast. Instead, I'm going to keep this chapter simple (just the way I like it).

Before I begin, let me say this: I am not a nutritionist. As I always say, your diet, like achieving fitness, is a progression. You need to incorporate small daily changes by making healthier choices. Sometimes diet information can be so overwhelming or confusing or contradictory that most people don't even know where to begin. For example, there are a lot of books promoting diets of no meat, no gluten, even no foods that are not right for your blood type! There is general truth in all of the studies to back up these theories, but you have to figure out what works best for you. I can tell you about my diet—just like I can tell you about my workout—and that might set you up for complete failure. How can I ask you to eat tuna if you hate fish? It seems as crazy as telling you to run 3 miles when you've never run 1 mile. No, you need to figure out what works for you. It can take time to discover the nutritional balance that best complements your life, plus those needs will likely change as time goes on.

I don't have a perfect diet, and every week I make goals for that time to progress toward making better food choices. And that's the approach you should take, too. Your job is to experiment with your options, eliminate what is holding you back, and execute to the best of your ability, week by week.

> The biggest remark I hear from overweight people is "But I don't eat that much!"
>
> Most people who are overweight don't eat. They skip breakfast or lunch and usually eat a heavy dinner. Or they snack on high-fat, high-sugar foods, drink their calories via fancy coffee drinks or sugary smoothies, and rarely cook their own meals. In order to lose weight, you have to eat. You have to eat more good food, consistently, throughout the day. If you look at most successful meal programs, the majority of them recommend eating small balanced meals throughout the day. It's not a secret. It's a science. Keep your metabolism churning and it will keep burning!

The Truth About Diets

There are a lot of misconceptions about what is healthy for you, but here are two guidelines I live by.

1. DIETING IS ABOUT PROGRESSION. Dieting is a progression, just like exercise. You don't go to the gym expecting to run a 7-minute mile! You practice every day, and you improve every week. For many (including myself), a 7-minute mile is extreme. It will probably take me a good year of hard training to be able to do that, but this type of perspective is what you need when you want to follow an extreme diet.

Dieting is the same way. When people talk about trying to lose weight, I tell them to *slowly* reduce their caloric intake. Going from eating 2,500-plus calories a day to eating just 1,200 is unhealthy and will be a major shock to your system. Not only is it unrealistic long term, but also your body will plateau and your weight-loss results stop because your metabolism will have shifted into starvation mode. Your system recalibrates and hoards your calories by metabolizing them at a slower rate. Also, I never recommend eating fewer than 1,200 calories a day. You need that many calories for energy and regular organ function!

2. EVERYTHING BOILS DOWN TO PORTION SIZE. The portion sizes in restaurants are *huge*. If you look at the caloric intake, even the salads could range from 600 to 1,000 calories! A cheeseburger twenty years ago was only 350 calories, but today the average is more than 550 calories for a fast-food cheeseburger. So, I often say the first step in your No More Excuses journey is to cut your portion sizes. Don't stop eating pizza if that's what you're used to eating. Just cut your portion size in half. When you reach a plateau, start substituting lower-calorie ingredients or make your own pizza.

Making small changes leads to bigger changes. Decreasing your portion size can mean dividing one meal into two! Sometimes I purchase a burrito and eat half for lunch and half for a snack. Often, I buy individually packed nuts because it's so easy to overeat them. Most of the time, I share whatever I'm consuming with my children. Sharing is caring, and cutting your portions will help with your bottom line!

The 30/30/30/10 Diet Plan

Macronutrients are the chemical compounds in the foods you consume. Each macronutrient provides calories to your body and serves different bodily functions. Get comfortable knowing the macronutrient profile of your favorite foods.

30 PERCENT PROTEIN

You need protein. Don't get me wrong; protein is essential to building and sustaining muscle. But protein is overrated.

When I say protein is overrated, I mean that there is often too much emphasis on a protein-based diet. You should most definitely eat protein, but you don't need to eat massive amounts of protein, especially in the form of animal products alone. Protein can also be found in dairy, nuts, and vegetables.

SEDENTARY VERSUS ACTIVE PROTEIN RECOMMENDATIONS

PERSON, SITUATION, AND GOALS	IDEAL DAILY PROTEIN INTAKE
Average healthy sedentary adult (male or female) that DOES NOT work out or have any related goals.	0.5 to 0.7 grams of protein per pound of body weight
Average healthy adult (male or female) that DOES some form of exercise regularly or is trying to engage in an activity program.	0.8 to 1.0 grams of protein per pound of body weight
Average healthy adult FEMALE whose primary goal is building muscle, increasing strength, losing fat, and improving physical performance.	1.0 to 1.2 grams of protein per pound of body weight
Average healthy adult MALE whose primary goal is building muscle, increasing strength, losing fat, and improving physical performance.	1.0 to 1.5 grams of protein per pound of body weight

HOW TO PORTION: There are many ways to consume protein outside of animal protein. Instead of pork, chicken, or beef, consider choosing fish, beans, tofu, eggs, or nuts. Incorporating protein requires you to have a good idea of what 25 to 30 grams of protein looks like. For example, most servings at restaurants provide 4 ounces of chicken breast or 25 grams of protein (approximately the size of your palm) in their meals. If you are highly active and eating an 1,800-calorie/day diet, then a minimum of 540 of your calories should be from protein, which is approximately 135 grams. You can achieve 135 grams of protein by consuming 35 grams at each primary meal and 15 grams at every snack time. Here are examples of common protein sources:

FOOD	PORTION	AMOUNT OF PROTEIN
Chicken Breast	4 ounces	25 grams
Salmon	4 ounces	30 grams
Turkey Patty	4 ounces	25 grams
Tuna	1 can	25 grams
Cottage Cheese	½ cup	25 grams
Almonds	½ cup	15 grams
Eggs	1 large	6 grams
Whole Milk	1 cup	8 grams
Tofu	1 cup	20 grams

30 PERCENT CARBOHYDRATES

Carbohydrates are used for energy. They are good for you! You need them to function. The problem with carbohydrates is that it's easy to consume too many, and sometimes they are from sources that are not so healthy. People don't realize that carbohydrates are everywhere, from the milk in a latte to the fruit in a smoothie to the beans in a burrito (and the tortilla and rice in the burrito, too)!

You should mainly be eating carbohydrates that are complex in nature. Carbohydrates are classified as either complex or simple and are divided by chemical structure and how quickly they digest and are absorbed in your body. Complex carbohydrates include high-fiber vegetables and whole grains and take longer to break down. Simple carbohydrates break down faster in your body and come in the form of fruits, honey, sugarcane, and syrups. While fruits and honey provide a lot of vitamins and minerals, refined sugar found in most processed foods not only offers little nutritional value but also promotes fat storage. Normally, refined sugar is just 20 percent of my total carbohydrate intake.

FOOD	PORTION	AMOUNT OF CARBOHYDRATES	AMOUNT OF SUGAR IN CARBOHYDRATES
Table Sugar	½ cup	49.99 grams	49.96 grams
Strawberry Jam	1 tablespoon	13 grams	12 grams
Honey	1 tablespoon	17 grams	17 grams

According to the Institute of Medicine, children and adults should consume at least 130 grams of carbohydrates per day. Determine your daily allowance by calculating 30 to 40 percent of your total caloric intake, and dividing it by 4. For example, if you eat a 2,000-calorie/day diet, shoot for 600 to 800 calories of carbohydrates or 150 to 200 grams of carbohydrates per day; and if you eat 2,500 calories a day, aim for 750 to 1,000 calories from carbohydrates or 188 to 250 grams of carbohydrates.

HOW TO PORTION: Carbohydrates are the easiest and most accessible macronutrient to consume. You can choose from whole wheat pasta, bread, crackers, cereal, oatmeal, or fruits. Depending on your overall goal, most people will eat a fistful of carbohydrates at each meal. Some of my favorites are:

FOOD	PORTION	AMOUNT OF CARBOHYDRATES
Brown Rice	½ cup	24 grams
Whole Wheat Bread	1 slice	24 grams
Oatmeal	1 cup	22 grams
Sweet Potato	1 cup	27 grams
Apple	1 medium	25 grams
Whole Wheat Tortilla	12-inch round	50 grams

30 PERCENT FAT

Fat has gotten such a bad rap. When I was younger, I was on a low-fat diet, purchasing mainly fat-free labeled foods. I avoided

FIBER IS YOUR KEY TO SUCCESS

A long time ago I wanted to write a book called *The Fiber Diet*. That's how important fiber is! Processed foods are often stripped of their nutrients, minerals, and fiber, which means that you feel less satisfied after eating. When you eat whole, unprocessed, and nearly raw foods, you are filling your belly with fiber, a type of carbohydrate that takes longer to digest and signals your brain that you're full.

There are two types of fiber—soluble and insoluble. *Soluble fiber,* found in legumes, oats, nuts, and fruits, dissolves in water. Imagine it meshing with your intestinal juices and turning into a gel that slows the movement of food through your system. *Insoluble fiber,* found in wheat, nuts, seeds, and vegetables, does not dissolve in water. It absorbs water as it moves through your system and has a bulking effect that promotes digestion. Unlike soluble fiber, insoluble fiber accelerates the movement of food through your system.

A high-fiber diet helps you detox your system by cleansing your colon regularly. Imagine eating three apples versus a bag of Skittles. They both have the same sugar content and calories, but the apple has more water and both types of fiber to create a

(continued on next page)

"bulking or gel-like effect" internally, making you feel full faster. It is recommended to consume 21 to 25 grams of fiber daily if you are a woman and 35 to 38 grams of fiber daily if you are a man. Fiber requirements slightly decrease as you age.

Some great sources of fiber are:

FOOD	PORTION	AMOUNT OF FIBER
Oat Bran (Raw)	1 ounce	12 grams
Fiber One Bran Cereal	½ cup	14 grams
All-Bran Cereal	½ cup	10 grams
Fiber One Chewy Bars	1 bar	9 grams
Black Beans (Cooked)	1 cup	15 grams
Garbanzo Beans (Cooked)	1 cup	12 grams
Kidney Beans (Cooked)	1 cup	16 grams
Raspberries (Raw)	1 cup	8 grams
Blueberries (Raw)	1 cup	4 grams

whole milk and nuts and instead ate fat-free saltine crackers and Skittles (because they had no fat) all the time! What I didn't realize then is that fat is good for you, especially the essential fats found in foods like salmon, olive oil, nuts, and avocados. Unsaturated fats are good for your brain, energy, and overall body function. You want the kind of fat that doesn't harden at room temperature. Paired with a balance of complex carbs and lean protein, you've got a winning diet!

The American Heart Association recommends eating between 25 and 35 percent of your total daily calories as fats, including fats in oils and fats in foods. Determine the number of grams of fat you need each day by calculating 30 percent of your total caloric intake, and dividing it by 9. For example, if you eat a 2,000-calorie/day diet, shoot for 600 calories of fats or 67 grams of fats per day; and if you eat 2,500 calories a day, aim for 750 calories from fats or 83 grams of fats.

COCONUT OIL

I don't often eat saturated fats, but when I do, I like my coconut oil. Studies show that it reduces cholesterol, improves heart health, strengthens immunity, promotes healthy brain function, and maintains youthful-looking skin! Not only does it help control blood sugar but it can also positively boost thyroid function and increase metabolism.

HOW TO PORTION: Compared with protein and carbohydrates, fats are more than double the calories gram for gram. Since fats are very dense in calories, consume a thumb-size serving at each meal. Another technique for fats found in nuts is to consume just a handful. Here are examples of portion sizes from my favorite unsaturated fats:

FOOD	PORTION	AMOUNT OF FAT
Peanuts	4 ounces	25 grams
Almonds	4 ounces	30 grams
Avocado	1 small	25 grams
Olive Oil	2 tablespoons	27 grams

10 PERCENT FLEXIBILITY

Since your activity expenditure, caloric needs, and physical goals fluctuate, you will need to be flexible about your eating plan. That's why I want you to customize the last 10 percent of your diet based on your level of activity. If you are very active, utilize that last 10 percent for additional carbohydrates for energy. If you are inactive, utilize the last 10 percent for additional protein for muscle, bones, and tissue repair. If you ate "perfectly" throughout the day but included a handful of jelly beans you grabbed at your coworker's desk or goldfish you ate with your child at the park, then call that your 10 percent and pat yourself on the back!

The last 10 percent is what makes the No More Excuses program flexible for your lifestyle. Remember, we are going for the long haul—it's the "this is it" eating plan that allows you to be imperfect while still losing weight. As long as you stay within your caloric intake, you will make progress and improve your health.

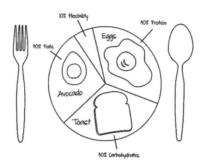

EXAMPLE OF MEAL PLANS BASED ON A 2,000-CALORIE/DAY DIET

MEAL	40/30/30	30/40/30	30/30/30/10
Breakfast	3 whole eggs, slice of toast, 1 tablespoon peanut butter	2 whole eggs, slice of toast, 1 tablespoon peanut butter, small apple	2 whole eggs, slice of toast, 1 tablespoon peanut butter, small low-fat latte
Snack	½ cup raw almonds	Small apple, ¼ cup almonds	⅓ cup honey-roasted almonds
Lunch	4 ounces grilled chicken, mixed greens salad with 2 to 3 tablespoons oil-based dressing	3 ounces grilled chicken, mixed greens salad with 2 tablespoons oil-based dressing, slice of wheat bread	4 ounces grilled chicken, mixed greens salad with 2 tablespoons oil-based dressing, handful of baked chips
Snack	⅔ cup hummus and 1 cup celery	⅓ cup hummus and ½ cup carrots	⅓ cup hummus with 1 cup pita chips
Dinner	6 ounces salmon, mixed vegetables	4 ounces salmon, mixed vegetables, ½ cup sweet potato	4 ounces salmon, mixed vegetables, ⅓ cup sweet potato, small piece of dark chocolate

Let's Talk Calories

A small calorie, or gram calorie as it is sometimes called, is the approximate amount of energy needed to raise the temperature of one gram of water by one degree Celsius. However, with regard to diets and nutrition, we talk of a large calorie, or kilogram calorie, which is the amount of energy needed to raise the temperature of one kilogram of water by one degree Celsius. That is, 1,000 small calories make up 1 large calorie. I know it sounds too scientific!

Basically, a calorie is potential energy. It is found in our foods in the form of protein, carbohydrates, and fats. These macronutrients are the three essentials that build muscle, provide energy, and maintain brain function. However, not all calories are created equal, for each macronutrient provides different calories per gram:

1 gram protein = 4 calories
1 gram carbohydrate = 4 calories
1 gram fat = 9 calories
1 gram alcohol = 7 calories

Every gram of food has different caloric values depending on its macronutrients. Following the 30/30/30/10 rule works well for me, as a physically active mother who still enjoys a glass of red wine, my children's peanut butter sandwich leftovers, and chocolate cravings—all while losing weight! Most days I use the remaining 10 percent for carbohydrates from the leftovers of my children's foods. Other days, when I am preparing to wear a bikini at the beach, I will utilize the last 10 percent for additional protein.

I believe the 30/30/30/10 approach is more flexible than traditional diets and reflects the average person's lifestyle. The more you stay consistent in an approach that is realistic, the more likely you will actually stick to the plan in the long term; this plan gives you room to indulge and alter your intake depending on your activity, cravings, and social events. This is a flexible No More Excuses formula that will help you lose weight yet not have to give up your favorite foods.

Meeting Your Caloric Needs

So how much food should you be eating? It depends on your body size and your weight-loss goal. Begin by testing your *basal metabolic rate* (BMR), which is a measure of how much fuel your body needs to lie in bed and do absolutely nothing. The most popular way to calculate your BMR is the *Harris-Benedict Equation*. While it is approximately accurate for the average person, it doesn't take into account your muscle composition, which can increase your metabolic output. Here's how to do the calculation:

1. **Calculate your BMR (basal metabolic rate):**
   - **Women:** BMR = 655 + (4.35 × weight in pounds) + (4.7 × height in inches) – (4.7 × age in years)
   - **Men:** BMR = 66 + (6.23 × weight in pounds) + (12.7 × height in inches) – (6.8 × age in years)

2. **Multiply your BMR by the appropriate activity factor, as follows:**
   - **Sedentary (little or no exercise):** BMR × 1.2
   - **Lightly active (light exercise/sports 1 to 3 days/week):** BMR × 1.375
   - **Moderately active (moderate exercise/sports 3 to 5 days/week):** BMR × 1.55
   - **Very active (hard exercise/sports 6 to 7 days a week):** BMR × 1.725
   - **Extra active (very hard exercise/sports and physical job or training twice a day):** BMR × 1.9

3. **Your final number is the approximate number of calories you need each day to maintain your weight.**

According to the Harris-Benedict Equation, my basal metabolic rate as a 33-year-old woman who is 5-foot-4 and weighs 125 pounds is figured as follows:

$655 + (4.35 \times 125 \text{ pounds}) + (4.7 \times 64 \text{ inches}) - (4.7 \times 33 \text{ years})$, or $(1,198.75) + (300.80) - (155.10) = 1,344 \text{ calories/day}$

This means that if I were lying in bed doing absolutely nothing, my body would need 1,344 calories daily just to sustain itself! When I add my activity level of moderate exercise 3 to 5 days per week (multiply by 1.55), my BMR changes to 2,083 calories per day!

I also have to keep in mind that 10 percent of the calories I consume (208 kilocalories out of 2,000 kilocalories total) are used to digest the foods I eat. This is called the *thermic effect of food* (TEF). That is, it takes calories to digest the calories you just ate! The digestion process includes when you bite, chew, and swallow, then process, transport, and metabolize the foods that pass through your system. The basic formula for determining your TEF is to multiply the total calories you eat by 10 percent.

So check how many calories you need, write down how much you are consuming, and start creating a 300- to 500-calorie deficit per day. A small deficit of just 300 to 500 calories will allow you to safely lose 2 to 3 pounds per week with exercise (more if you're heavier). You can create this small change by eating half the foot-long sandwich or eliminating the fancy coffee drink every morning. By changing your portion sizes or eliminating an entire snack, you can lose weight and do it without drastically changing your diet.

Get to know how many calories are in the foods you commonly eat. Know them off the top of your head! For example, do you know how many calories are in an apple, a slice of bread, a small cheeseburger, or one cookie? I carried a small calorie book and used a calorie phone app to help me determine how many calories are in foods until I started remembering the numbers, then I used the app for less common foods.

Put It All Together

Here are the steps for making your diet guidelines.

1. **Figure out your BMR + activity level + TEF.**
2. **Write down your current food intake (without dieting) and calculate the calories.**
3. **Identify where you can create a 300- to 500-calorie deficit.**
4. **Start decreasing your portion sizes.**
5. **Begin focusing on eating five small meals a day.**
6. **Follow the 30/30/30/10 meal plan by focusing on your three macronutrients: lean protein, complex carbohydrates, and unsaturated fats.**
7. **Apply the 80:20 principle by enjoying one or two planned treat meals weekly.**
8. **Create a S.P.E.E.D. strategy and start executing. If you aren't delivering your best results, set new goals by altering your caloric intake, switching your macronutrient profile, or modifying your activity level.**

These changes will yield results, but your weight-loss efforts will reach plateaus. At those points, you will have to change your diet to keep your body and metabolism guessing. I will make recommendations for doing this in later chapters. For now, let's put these pieces together.

THREE MEAL PLAN OPTIONS

Each person should consume a balanced macronutrient diet of 30/30/30/10, and alter it depending on the individual's needs. There is a lot of flexibility with the No More Excuses diet plan, allowing you to switch up your macronutrient profile throughout each meal. Here are some options for good No More Excuses diet plans.

OPTION 1: BALANCED DIET

BREAKFAST	SNACK	LUNCH	SNACK	DINNER
30/30/30/10	30/30/30/10	30/30/30/10	30/30/30/10	30/30/30/10

EXAMPLE OF BALANCED MACRONUTRIENT PROFILE BASED ON A 2,000-CALORIE/DAY DIET

MACRONUTRIENT	CALORIES	GRAMS
Protein	600 calories	150 grams
Carbohydrates	600 calories	150 grams
Fats	600 calories	66 grams
Flexibility	200 calories	*Varies by macronutrient*

Meal Examples

BREAKFAST: turkey bacon, eggs, sliced wheat bread, and some butter

SNACK: apple, peanut butter

LUNCH: tuna salad open-faced whole wheat sandwich with veggie chips

SNACK: leftover tuna salad and wheat crackers

DINNER: chicken marsala, rice pilaf, asparagus (and perhaps some dark chocolate)

OPTION 2: FAT-LOSS DIET

BREAKFAST	SNACK	LUNCH	SNACK	DINNER
40/30/30	40/30/30	40/30/30	40/30/30	40/30/30

EXAMPLE OF FAT-LOSS MACRONUTRIENT PROFILE BASED ON A 2,000-CALORIE/DAY DIET

MACRONUTRIENT	CALORIES	GRAMS
Protein	800 calories	200 grams
Carbohydrates	600 calories	150 grams
Fats	600 calories	66 grams

Meal Examples

BREAKFAST: egg white vegetable omelet with avocado and portion of oatmeal

SNACK: almonds

LUNCH: grilled chicken salad

SNACK: celery and peanut butter

DINNER: steak and mixed vegetables

OPTION 3: ACTIVE LIFESTYLE DIET

BREAKFAST	SNACK	LUNCH	SNACK	DINNER
30/40/30	30/40/30	30/40/30	30/40/30	30/40/30

EXAMPLE OF ACTIVE MACRONUTRIENT PROFILE BASED ON A 2,000-CALORIE/DAY DIET

MACRONUTRIENT	CALORIES	GRAMS
Protein	600 calories	150 grams
Carbohydrates	800 calories	200 grams
Fats	600 calories	66 grams

Meal Examples

BREAKFAST: eggs and wheat waffles with syrup

SNACK: fruit smoothie of berries, banana, milk, and flaxseed

LUNCH: turkey burger on whole wheat bun

SNACK: trail mix

DINNER: whole wheat spaghetti, marinara sauce, and lean beef meatballs

You can't follow "generic" diet programs because they do not take into account your personal situation or tastes. For those trying to eat only chicken and broccoli all day, you know how tough it is when you prefer ethnic foods. What do you do if you hate chicken? Or if you're allergic to nuts? You have to do what's best for *you,* which means finding the better options among what you like to eat. For instance, if you like to eat pizza, start seeking healthier pizza recipes and cut back on your cookie eating. If you want to stick to a healthy program for the long term, you have to create your own plan, not use someone else's.

At this point, you have your S.P.E.E.D. strategy, your baseline measurements, your action calendar, weekly workout plan, meal plan, and excuse-busting tactics. These upcoming months won't always be easy, but don't get frustrated! If you run into challenges, turn the page to find my best troubleshooting techniques!

PART 3

S.T.R.I.V.E.

Seek Out Reasons

Tackle the Problem

Reflect on Your Game Plan

Revisit Your **I**ntentions

Value the Lesson

Emerge with a New Attitude

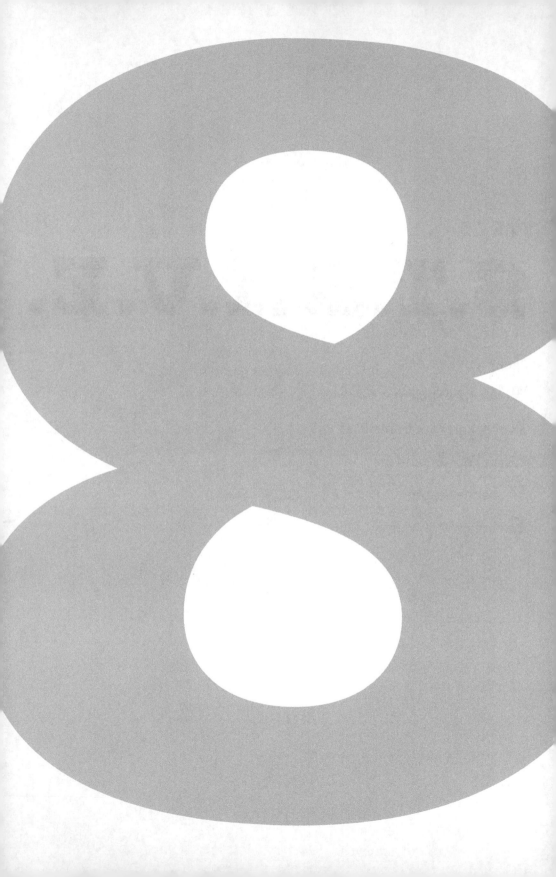

S.T.R.I.V.E. TOWARD CONTINUED SUCCESS

The S.T.R.I.V.E. model is here for you when life's trials start kicking in. These generally come along after the initial kickoff and honeymoon. You're settling into the reality of your new commitment. You're hungry, you're sore, and you're mentally drained from making conscious choices to perform healthy acts on a daily basis. How do you keep going?

This is when you must **S**eek out reasons you're not seeing results, **T**ackle the problem, **R**eflect on your game plan, revisit your **I**ntentions, **V**alue the lesson, and **E**merge with a new attitude. S.T.R.I.V.E. helps you review your program in a concise way so you can troubleshoot to get through the emotional trials and bust through the excuses. It's the tool that will carry you over your hurdles and help you stay focused, no matter what life throws at you.

You've set your goals; you're in execution mode, and you are striving to become your very best. The ultimate goal in designing any fitness program is to become master of your own body. But to do so, you must know your weaknesses, your strengths, your motivations, your patterns, and your life routine. You should be paying attention to what foods make you tired, what exercises make you sore, and what times you are motivated to train, prepare, and reflect. No one is perfect, which is why mastering your body is a continuous journey experienced only through serious reflection.

The path to wellness will take you on this journey for the rest of your life. It's a hard truth to swallow: Being healthy today doesn't mean you won't struggle tomorrow. Fortunately, the opposite is true, too: If you're struggling with your health or weight today, tomorrow is an opportunity to see things improve!

Life unfolds in seasons, and there will be times when you grow, peak, and rest. Understanding the rhythm of your life will help you master your efforts as you continue to grow and evolve in personal wellness, physical health, and spiritual satisfaction. Striving to become better physically, personally, and professionally requires you to challenge yourself, though. And the only way to challenge yourself is to change your daily habits. Creating successful habits requires small, conscious efforts, so you won't fry your mental machinery. But how do you do this? How do you stay successful? How do you keep going? How do you avoid burning out? How do you keep from giving up?

You keep striving.

Troubleshoot Your Struggle

No matter how good your intentions were at the start of the program, it's likely that by now something has happened that made you falter. Negative people are getting under your skin. Special events or holidays have come along to disrupt your routine and kill your motivation. Setbacks will happen and frustrations will kick in. I know it; I've been there. I've injured my ankle, shoulder, and back a few times. I've dealt with depression, disordered eating, and six years in a row of the "terrible twos." But you cannot wait for things to be going well to make positive changes in your life.

Arianna Huffington, a successful journalist, political scientist, and media entrepreneur, once said, "You can't wait for things to be going well to start thriving." It's great to have a plan and execute with perfect precision. But in between our winning shots is real life, where the excuses lurk around every corner and small setbacks feel like large failures. We are all on a journey, and there is no real end to the journey toward good health, until the day you depart this world.

So embrace the fact that this ride is going to have bumps. You need to maintain your drive to succeed. So, let's start our engines and S.T.R.I.V.E. for success!

SEEK OUT REASONS THINGS AREN'T WORKING

If you're not seeing the results you want, it's time to seek the reasons why. Once a week, usually on Sundays, I take a step back and really look at what's going on. It's important to see what you're doing—both right and wrong—so you can efficiently plan your upcoming week. The only way to create a solution is to seek the problem.

During my post-pregnancy weight loss, I hit a plateau. Though I was exercising four or five times a week and eating well, I didn't get physical results for nearly a month. So, I had to *seek* the reason for my setback. I determined my diet needed to be changed. I was working out intensely while maintaining a caloric deficit, but I was not seeing results. I did more research on my basal metabolic rate (BMR) and recalculated how many calories I should healthfully consume while exercising and still lose weight. Of course, this caloric number was adjusted depending on whether I was nursing, sick, or training for a long charity run. I realized I didn't have enough caloric variation on active days and I felt my energy plummeting from lack of fuel. I had a lightbulb moment when I realized that, in order to get off this plateau, I needed to challenge not only my muscles but my metabolism as well!

I altered my intake to reflect my greater activity levels and I challenged my metabolism by increasing my caloric intake. It was startling to realize I was on a weight-loss plateau possibly because I had not been eating enough! So ask yourself: Are you losing weight? Are you missing workouts? Are you following your program rules 100 percent? Are you writing down everything you eat? To create change, something has to be changed. You can't continue doing similar actions weekly and expect different results.

TACKLE THE PROBLEM

Once you've discovered why you're not making progress, tackle the challenge head-on. Don't be discouraged or daunted by the fact that you've discovered an obstacle; start finding your way around it! Take on the problem aggressively and assertively, and with all your mental might. Grab hold of this problem and start controlling it—after all, this problem is preventing you from getting to the next level in your fitness goals. So control it, and believe me when I tell you that you can change it!

While losing the baby weight after pregnancy, I ate a healthy diet and exercised daily. I enjoyed doing Zumba, taking kickboxing classes, and going for the occasional run. Despite what I did,

I couldn't regain a strong midsection, even though I would log sometimes a thousand sit-ups in one day! When I sought the reasons I wasn't becoming more "toned," I discovered the importance of strength training. Because I was a "scale watcher" the idea of building muscle was a little scary to me. Gaining muscle mass often means you need to let go of the number on the scale, however, because a pound of muscle is much smaller than a pound of fat—it's tighter and denser. When I knew I wouldn't turn into a bodybuilder, I became comfortable lifting light weights.

It was a scary process to walk onto the gym floor, over to the free-weights section, and hear the clinking of iron and smell the rubber, sweat, and bad cologne. It was emotionally tougher to stand next to young women who have never had a child or seemed to be athletically gifted (another excuse I gave myself). Nevertheless, I needed to tackle the matter and start educating myself about this activity. I gained confidence daily by setting small, short-term goals and reading about new exercises on the Internet while I was nursing or flipping through fitness magazines while waiting in line at the grocery store. Whatever obstacle you want to resolve, the first step is to tackle it head-on and create a game plan.

REFLECT ON YOUR PLAN

Reflection is a cornerstone of your constructed new world. Whether you are failing or succeeding in your efforts, it's important to be aware every step along the journey. Reflection is not about feeling guilty or beating yourself up; it's just being aware of *why* you're not progressing on schedule. Its result is to give yourself permission to consider *how* to change your course so as to reach that success. For example, if my goal is to develop better abdominal muscles, I need to change my game plan so as to lose 5 pounds so I can uncover my toned abs.

So reflect on your plan and break it apart. If your goal is to get leaner, could you start incorporating an extra day of weights? If you are constantly missing your workouts, can you schedule your exercise for a different time of day? If you need more personal accountability or knowledge, can you enlist the help of a trainer or friend? What do you plan to do?

Most recently I was preparing for a fitness event, so I was running two to four miles daily. However, I fell on concrete and injured my neck and back. It was a huge blow to my progress and it prevented me from training for a couple weeks. Instead of dwelling on my anger and getting frustrated, I reflected on this new challenge to stay fit and changed my game plan. I focused on eating healthier foods and I created a caloric deficit and macronutrient profile to reflect my lowered activity level. Instead of running, I scheduled various therapies and incorporated rest into my program to recover from the injury. So, just because you have a setback, that does not mean the program stops. The program is about living your healthiest life in the circumstances in which you are living today. Remember that.

REVIEW YOUR INTENTIONS

Your intention is the seed your mind plants before you develop your action plans. When you need more energy to pursue your goal, you must look at the present moment and ask yourself, *Why does this effort matter so much to me? What was my intention when I decided to take the first step in changing my life? Do I want to impress family at an upcoming reunion? Do I want to feel comfortable in tank tops and shorts during the summer? Do I want to extend my life span? Was I pre-diabetic or did a family member just die from heart disease?*

Reaching long-term goals requires you to set short-term goals. Setting short-term goals will keep you motivated because you are focusing on a reachable target. You wake up each day and state your intention. You think about your action and find your motivation to complete it.

My ultimate goal is to feel fit and be healthy for my husband and children. Vanity also plays a big role in my efforts: I know that I want to look great in a cocktail dress and feel toned in a bikini! But when life becomes busy and I keep finding my hand in the cookie jar, I always think about why staying disciplined is so important. Sometimes a small motivator is enough to get me back on track: *Do I want to call off the race? Do I want to return that dress?* Other times, I can renew my intention by thinking about the big picture: *What will happen to my health if I slack off?* It's easy to get lost in the business of just getting through each day, but that's why it is so important to regularly check in with your goals and remind yourself what they are all about.

VALUE THE LESSONS LEARNED

When you look for value in every moment, you start seeing opportunities and possibilities. Maybe you don't have spousal support, a gym membership, a large grocery budget, or a babysitter, but what you do have is the ability to choose your attitude. Do not focus on the things you don't have—that will only lead you to spend more energy on why you can't do what you want rather than on working to get it. No matter what your circumstances, it is within your power to arrange your life around the things that are most important to you. Realize that *it is possible to get the life you want.* Every day, life's changes and challenges shift. Don't dwell on the possibility that things might be easier if your life were different; focus on the way your life is now and appreciate your indelible spirit and unwillingness to give up.

Time is your most valuable commodity. Finding enough time is a challenge for everyone, including myself. As a busy working wife and mother, I rarely have time to relax or feel that I'm doing something for myself. Even though my schedule is back-to-back with obligations, errands, sports practices, and work right now, I know that life will change. My kids will get older, I will get older, and I don't want to look back wishing I had valued all my moments a little more. I want to make sure that every action I take brings value to my life. Working out brings value. Playing at the park with my kids brings value. Giving back to my community brings value. Developing relationships brings value.

Strive to live a valuable life. Slow down and be deliberate about who you are and where you are going in life. Be mindful of your priorities and ensure that your values, including your thoughts, actions, and results, all align. When your moments start to mean something, you've gained a force that drives you in a purposeful direction.

EMERGE WITH A NEW ATTITUDE

It's not easy to identify a dream and go for it—let's face it, most people give up. Most people don't dig deep, mentally and spiritually, to uncover the root of the struggle. To succeed, you need to seek the problem, tackle it with a plan, reflect on the plan, keep sight of your intentions, value the moment, and emerge with renewed vigor.

Your priorities will change with time; your intentions will change, too. Your body and mind will most definitely change. In the process, you must always keep *striving* to get the most out of your time and your efforts. S.T.R.I.V.E. is not about pushing yourself harder in the same direction or whipping yourself into a short-term frenzy of activity; this is about making sure that you are actively engaged and conscious of what your goals are—and living by them each day.

Develop a New Strategy

With careful observation of your body and your habits, you will find a way to climb out of any rut and see results. Do not feel frustrated that you hit a roadblock. Do not get discouraged, and above all do NOT quit. The health, the body, and the life you want are within your reach—all you have to do is S.T.R.I.V.E. to grab them!

Take out a pen and paper and start a new S.P.E.E.D. strategy, considering how you can tweak the routine to keep your motivation high. Write down your new goals, create a new action plan, and emerge as a refreshed No More Excuses person. You can do this. You are capable of overcoming challenges, and you will create your best body. It all begins with a thought and it proceeds with an action.

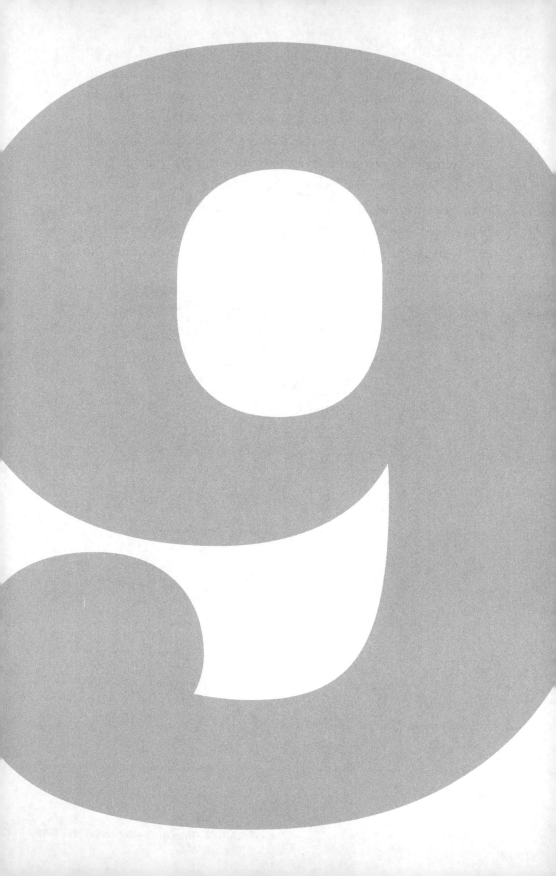

WHAT'S YOUR EXCUSE?

It is so easy to get distracted from our goals. We can get discouraged when something's not working fast enough, or we get cocky when we start seeing results. But it doesn't have to be that way! And right now, today, you have a chance to make a new commitment to yourself and your body, no matter what else is happening in your life. In this chapter, we look at the most common excuses that prevent so many of us from having the lives and the bodies we want. Believe me, I know how real many of these situations can feel—I've been there! But nothing is more important than good health, and it's time right now to make a new commitment to yourself.

I recently received an email from a woman who said she continued to exercise and eat healthy despite gaining weight and undergoing depression from her treatment for breast cancer. She expressed feeling weak, helpless, and defeated on a daily basis. She had plenty of reasons to let herself off the hook, but she chose to exercise, eat healthy, and strive toward health.

A friend in her thirties is suffering from congestive heart failure, diabetes, and end-stage renal disease. She works full time as the primary breadwinner for her family of four, and yet spends 12 hours a week in the dialysis chair. Despite her challenges she is focusing on positive actions and has lost 30 pounds in 12 weeks. She recently posted, "If anyone is overweight, out of shape, and mad about it, remember that you have a choice. You can choose to remain the way you are or put the work in and change your lot in life. I did."

A single working mother of four children shared with me her struggle to get into shape. I was impressed by her vigilance, ability, and creativity to incorporate exercise into her hectic schedule while managing expenses on her own. One of my closest girlfriends battled polycystic ovarian syndrome, a hormonal imbalance that affects 5 million women in America. Although weight gain was one of her symptoms, she was able to lose weight, take supplements to balance her hormones, and is now a marathon runner.

We can take so much hope from such stories. These women had legitimate excuses for giving in, but they believed they could improve their lives, and they succeeded in doing so.

For every excuse you have, there is a way to overcome it. But you have to want to do it and believe that you *can* do it. Believe that you can reach your highest potential. Believe that every obstacle is a test of how badly you want to achieve your best body. And believe that you are stronger than those obstacles and tests. Success doesn't come easily, and it only serves those who are mentally and physically willing to do the work that brings results.

So let's bust those excuses right now. A successful fitness lifestyle requires a goal, a plan, a deadline, and a desire. This desire is the energy that propels you forward. Yes, let's blast these excuses off the road toward your fitness future.

Excuse #1: I Don't Have Time

You need to schedule your workouts the same way you schedule your doctors' appointments, work meetings, and family meals. Your exercise needs to be a planned appointment at least three days a week for a minimum of 30 minutes each time. Take a good look at your schedule and figure out what you are doing on an hour-by-hour basis. The most opportune times to incorporate a workout are in the morning, during your lunch break, or directly after work. Some people get their training done close to bedtime, but for most people, exercising late in the day impedes quality sleep. So you have to figure out what works for you.

My best advice is to exercise right when you get up in the morning. The morning is a time when you can't think yourself out of working out. Set your alarm clock, have your workout clothes ready—perhaps even sleep in them—so that all you have to do is brush your teeth and start exercising. The energy boost that you will feel from getting your heart pumping at the beginning of your day will make it worth rising a little earlier.

When I first had my children, I worked out right after I nursed my infant at 5 AM. I put on my running shoes and hopped on my treadmill for 30 minutes. Sometimes I ran outside or performed a workout DVD. Whatever I did, I made sure it was done in the morning when my head and body were fresh; once the boys woke up, all of my energy was focused on caretaking, cleaning, cooking, working, and surviving the daily hustle.

But time is one of your most valuable assets, and you need to be able to efficiently and effectively utilize it. You have to eliminate things that waste your time. There is definitely nothing wrong with playing video games, watching TV, or surfing the Internet; everybody needs a mental break! But while half an hour of online shopping or watching an episode of your favorite show can be a good way to unwind, you can't spend hours vegging out in front of a screen if you want to have a healthy life.

Tally up how long it takes to perform your tasks and see how you can get them done faster by using focus and organization. Write down your task list and create appointments for each, including exercise! Be realistic about your schedule and figure out the best, uninterrupted, flow times to perform your daily tasks.

Flow times are when you are most efficient. For example, it takes me 30 minutes to fold and put away four loads of laundry, but if I'm playing with my phone or trying to complete this task at a bad time—such as when the boys are awake—then it takes me closer to an hour. Sometimes you can't avoid having to complete certain tasks at inconvenient times, but it's important to be aware of when you are able to do each kind of work.

Lastly, when you lack time, always remember that your success is 80 percent diet and 20 percent exercise. So if you can't get the additional 30 to 60 minutes of exercise in your day, this means you need to be more vigilant about your intake. Eating healthy doesn't require additional time; it just demands that you choose healthier options when eating.

HOW TO BUST THE EXCUSE

Write down your goals every evening, and plan out your next day. For each day, block out one 30-minute interval for some kind of heart-pumping exercise, choosing different times each day of the week: If you usually exercise after work, try setting your alarm earlier; if you always promise to wake up early but find yourself hitting the snooze button, schedule a workout during your lunch break; if mornings are too hectic for you, find a way to get in a quick session before your dinnertime. Trying out different times for your workout will help you settle on the best fit with your schedule. Having "made an appointment with your exercise" will remind you that your health is just as important as that meeting, doctor's appointment, or scheduled pickup.

Excuse #2: Eating Healthy Is So Expensive

Anyone who argues that healthy eating isn't expensive hasn't looked at a fast-food menu lately (and yes, I sometimes find myself at a drive-through!). Trust me, I get it: Purchasing fresh vegetables and fruits seems more expensive than buying a box of fruit snacks on clearance. But don't lose hope. If you start recognizing what defines real food, you will begin shopping wisely, and I promise you that you will actually reduce the amount of money you're spending on food.

You have to understand that your health is an investment worth making. When you exercise and eat nutritious foods, you are investing in a long and healthy life. Like any goal worth striving for, it will take planning so that you invest in that body to take you through this life. While it requires extra effort to consume nutritious foods, it costs a lot more to deal with health problems, including prescription pills you'll need in the future. According to a study conducted by the Brookings Institute, obesity directly results in increased medical spending. Since excess weight is linked to serious health conditions such as type 2 diabetes, coronary heart disease, stroke, and hypertension, obese patients have 105 percent higher prescription costs and 39 percent higher primary care costs.

Eating healthy is a good investment for the long haul, and it is affordable if you just start making some strategic choices about where you get your food. Most processed foods are laden with trans fats, salt, additives, food coloring, and highly addictive ingredients like high fructose corn syrup. Not only are processed foods stripped of most of their nutritional value, but they are also void of fiber, the roughage found in carbohydrates that satisfies your hunger and triggers your brain to notify you that your stomach is full. So even if you get a great price on chips, cookies, fruit snacks, and frozen dinners because they were all on sale, you will end up eating more of them at a time because these "foods" lack nutritional value and fiber. You will wind up spending much more money because the food you're buying doesn't leave you feeling satisfied.

There are ways to integrate healthy foods into your diet without breaking the bank. So start buying the foods that will give you more bang for your grocery buck. Here are some quick tips:

1. **For large items like poultry, fish, and beef, buy in bulk when you see discounts and store them in your freezer.**

2. **You can lower your grocery bill by purchasing seasonal fruits and vegetables.** When you buy a watermelon in the winter, it will cost more than if you purchase it during the summer.

3. **Never underestimate the benefits of using coupons.** Every little bit saved adds up. You can find coupons online, in newspapers, and on direct mailers in your mailbox. With just a few minutes of advanced planning, you can save big this way.

4. **For your vegetables and fruits, local farmers' markets often have good prices on fresh vegetables.** Not only can you develop a relationship with your local farmers, but you can also bargain for reduced prices, especially if you go near closing time and get fruits that are more ripe.

5. **If you can't buy fresh vegetables, consider buying them frozen.** As soon as a fruit or vegetable is plucked, it loses nutritional and mineral value. When it's frozen immediately after harvest, the nutrients are locked in. Most often, too, there are no additives, making frozen food as healthy as its fresh counterpart.

6. **Eat more nuts.** If you are not allergic, nuts are a great way to incorporate healthy fats, fiber, and protein. They are high in cal-

ories, but offer a lot of nutritional value. They keep well, too; put them in the freezer to extend their shelf life.

7. **Stock up on canned foods.** While canned chicken, tuna, and salmon aren't the freshest choice, they offer a great alternative when you have a tight budget. If you go this route, check the nutrition label to make sure the option you've chosen is packed in water and do your best to choose the ones with the smallest amount of added sodium. Chicken and tuna sandwiches are great lunch options!

Purchasing organic fruits and vegetables can be pricey, so reserve your purchases of the organics for foods that normally have the highest concentrations of pesticides. The "Dirty Dozen" is an annual list of foods by the Environmental Working Group (EWG) that analyzes Department of Agriculture data about pesticide residue and ranks foods based on how much each food has. You can greatly reduce your pesticide exposure if you stick to organic versions of the following:

Apples	Nectarines (imported)
Celery	Peaches
Cherry tomatoes	Potatoes
Cucumbers	Spinach
Grapes	Strawberries
Hot peppers	Sweet bell peppers

Create a garden of your own if you have the space. You can grow herbs from seed; you can plant a dwarf or semi-dwarf fruit tree that will yield fruit in a couple of years. Green beans, tomatoes, lettuce, spinach, peppers, and zucchini are all easily grown in a backyard garden and require little care. If you have limited garden space, consider setting up a tower or vertical

(continued on next page)

garden, or even an herb garden in pots on a kitchen windowsill. You don't have to be too ambitious in growing your own food. By growing a couple of types of fruits and/or vegetables, you can cut your grocery costs.

Remember, your health is your life, and eating healthy foods is a crucial step toward living a long and enjoyable life. So consider the trade-offs; for example, do you need to have 150 cable channels, or could you choose a less expensive package and put the extra $30 toward a healthier grocery cart? Is it better to spend an extra $10 on high-quality foods or thousands of dollars on a coronary artery bypass? You choose.

HOW TO BUST THE EXCUSE

Maybe you've heard the saying "Health Is Wealth." It's true! Your health should be treated as an investment that can be affordable on any budget if you put your mind to it. If the cost of food is deterring you from achieving your best body, then it's time to start making changes. Review your personal budget and assess how much you're spending on different kinds of food. Clean out your freezer and make room for bulk meats that go on sale. Research your local farmers' markets and look in your local paper or online for weekly discounts. Cut back if you are eating out more than two meals per week; not only could you be saving money but you can never be sure of what ingredients go into your takeout or restaurant meals.

Excuse #3: I Don't Have a Gym

Working out doesn't require a gym. In fact, it doesn't even require a workout video or training shoes! When I became a mother, I started a free "mom group" in my local park. My eldest son was too young for me to take along to the gym and it was tough for me to leave him because I was nursing. So the other moms and I worked out at the park, performing body-weight exercises like step-ups, push-ups, tricep dips, squats, crunches, and planks while we kept an eye on our kids. Talk about multitasking!

All you need is a little knowledge about how your body works (which I cover in Chapter 6). Keep reading and you'll find all the resources you need to turn any space—your bedroom, a public park, even where you work—into a place where you can get in a workout!

HOW TO BUST THE EXCUSE

Pick a corner in your house and designate that as your workout space. This can be in the living room in front of the TV (where you exercise following a DVD) or in your garage where you placed your elliptical. Find a space and take your time to furnish it with your No More Excuses fitness tools. You can find inexpensive videos and workout equipment online, at consignment stores, and at garage sales. Wait for new workout DVDs and/or dumbbells, resistance bands, medicine balls, and foam rollers to go on sale, then buy what you need. Even my tiny home gym took years to build. I asked for fitness equipment on my holidays and birthdays and eyed garage sales for cardio equipment. You don't have to spend any money to work out—all you need to do is create a small space for your "me time" and take a little bit of every day to make your fitness goals happen.

Excuse #4: I Don't Have Any Support

A successful environment includes the people in your world, not just keeping a healthful pantry and having access to a gym membership. Not having support for your goals can be damaging, especially when your schedule and life are tied to others.

How do you overcome the discomfort of always explaining and showcasing your healthy lifestyle choices? It's not easy skipping happy hour because you have a date at the gym. It's difficult to order seltzer with lemon when your friends are buying a round of cocktails. It's not easy going to bed early because you're prioritizing sleep and are waking the next day to train. Look, fitness isn't about avoiding everything unhealthy, and of course you should celebrate and enjoy special occasions. But if you want to change your life, you need to be selective about when you splurge, and you have to be firm about living by your priorities, even when people are trying to coax you to do something else.

But stand strong! It's an amazing thing to keep your eyes on the prize, and nobody should make you feel embarrassed or ashamed of sticking to your goals. There will always be people who look at you and say "you're fine the way you are" or who encourage you to partake in poor habits because "one splurge won't hurt." There may be family members who insist you have a second serving of food, or who make you feel bad for not sampling the macaroni and cheese they proudly cooked. It might feel awkward at first, but you need to stay strong with your message to the world about your priorities. Gradually people will realize that your new habits are helping you become the best version of yourself that you can be. And if they are truly people worth having in your life, they will celebrate that with you!

It's not easy saying no to food, especially when it comes from a family member, but here are five graceful ways to say no to an undesired splurge:

1. Express that you are full because you already ate.

2. Tell them you are allergic to an ingredient.

3. Request they pack it up for you to take to go.

4. Say you've had recent stomach/digestive issues.

5. Be honest and tell them about your new eating plan.

Now, of course, not everyone is going to jump on your healthy-living bandwagon right away. That's okay; you don't need everyone to be on the same healthy page as you. However, you will need three key people to help you transition into your No More Excuses lifestyle.

- First, find a mentor who can steer you in the right direction. This person can be someone who is passionate about health and fitness, works in the health industry, or has succeeded at maintaining a healthy No More Excuses lifestyle. (You could also consider me your mentor, since my best advice is in this book!) Your mentor will guide you through the process as someone who has walked your path. He or she understands the real struggle in finding your confidence, revealing your strength, and educating yourself to sort out the facts from the myths around health and fitness. Approach this person by acknowledging his or her success and asking for top advice in getting in shape. See if you can continue asking health questions and use the individual as a role model in this No More Excuses journey. Your mentor should be someone you feel comfortable asking for advice and should be able to provide you with the tools needed to get to your destination, including dealing with excuses that have prevented your success in the past.

- Next, choose your supporter. You need a cheerleader—someone who will say "You can do this!" Having a supporter, whether it's a partner, a friend, or an online acquaintance, will keep you motivated. This person won't make you feel bad for rejecting his or her homemade cookies or try to persuade you to ditch the gym and make other plans. Find someone to whom you can freely send selfies of your progress or meal pictures—someone who makes you feel comfortable enough to discuss your challenging and triumphant days. Choose your supporter by calling to task a person online or in person to be your "go to" during your No More Excuses journey. Tell the individual that you appreciate his or her role in your life and know that one of that person's best qualities is being honest, encouraging, and caring. Ask if you can rely on that person for support, and thank him or her for playing an ongoing positive role in your life.

- Lastly, enlist a follower. Life is about give-and-take—it's about balance. So in order to receive, you must also give. Find someone whom you can inspire, motivate, and guide. Think of the friend who is struggling to balance her work, family, and fitness. Consider the family member who is struggling with self-confidence. Think about a person who has lost hope after undergoing multiple diets or medical ailments. Becoming a role model creates a level of personal and social responsibility; knowing that someone is counting on you to set a good example is a great way to hold yourself accountable. In helping others, you are in essence helping yourself. Seek a follower by telling that person you are on this journey and looking for people who will join you. Don't make the individual think you pity him or her; rather, let the person know you are on this journey to becoming healthier and ask if he or she wants to come along. Keep each other accountable and check in every week.

Sometimes, support comes from places outside your inner circle. Perhaps a coworker commits to running with you every lunch hour or an online friend swaps her fitness goals, recipes, challenges, and achievements. If you lack support, consider connecting with people who are like-minded online and in fitness groups in your area. Many cities have running clubs, "mom groups," or other meet-up groups that focus on recreational fitness activities.

For many people, support within your immediate group isn't instant. After all, the reason you are overweight is most likely your overall environment, including your family and friends who engage in unhealthy habits with you. But you don't have to be alone in trying to get healthy! If you feel frustrated, find someone who will partner with you in this effort to be healthy. This comforting energy can be found in person or online. As long as you feel you're not alone in this process, you will gather the mental strength to keep moving forward. Eventually, people within your circle will see your progress and seek guidance when they are ready to make changes.

HOW TO BUST THE EXCUSE

Talk to your family and close friends first. Explain what you're trying to do, and tell them how they can help you. Initiate the conversation by telling them how excited you are about choosing a healthier lifestyle. Tell them you appreciate their important role in your life and hope they can be supportive of you on this challenging journey. Look through your Facebook friends and notice the ones who enjoy posting their run times and fitspiration posters. Send them a message and collaborate on how to keep each other accountable.

If you aren't able to find the team you want, get online and start researching groups. There are online support groups and local recreational fitness groups. If you search Noexcusemom.com and Meetup.com, you will find local groups that focus on connecting people through fitness.

Excuse #5: I'm Too Tired

Energy drinks have grown into a $9-billion industry. Checkout stands are loaded with tiny liquid-filled energy bottles. Coffee shops are stationed at every street corner. People are looking for something to wake themselves up, give them endurance, and make them active. What people don't seem to realize is that seeking external sources of energy is a short-term solution to a problem they can fix naturally and internally.

It's hard to work out, plan meals, and be efficient if you have no energy. When you have several priorities pulling you in different directions, it's difficult to force yourself to do one more thing, like work out. For many, working out sounds just like that: work! It's another thing on your to-do list that seemingly strips you of energy that you already lack.

But while it might not feel this way right away, exercise actually gives you more energy. Exercise gets your blood circulating and muscles moving, creating happy hormones—endorphins—that boost your self-esteem and make you energetic and aware. Additionally, nourishing your body with foods that are nutrient and mineral rich is another way of boosting your energy, in a healthier, longer lasting way than with a quick shot of caffeine.

Being too tired to do what's best for your body is a self-perpetuating cycle, so let's break it now, together! Check out the following list of energy-boosting techniques, and pick five to start integrating into your life today. You won't believe how amazing you will feel.

1. MOVE.

When you're feeling drowsy, wake up your body with a little movement! Getting your muscles engaged elevates your endorphins (your happy hormones), promotes blood flow, and decreases stress and anxiety. Try taking a power walk, performing a set of lunges or squats, doing some jumping jacks, or performing another set of movements to activate your body.

2. SIT UP STRAIGHT.

Posture not only enables you to breathe properly but as a result of better breathing, you also can concentrate better because more oxygen is getting to the brain. See the Appendix for more tips on improving your posture.

3. ELONGATE YOUR BODY AND STRETCH.
Stretching improves circulation because it helps blood flow to the muscles. Studies have shown that it also decreases blood pressure and improves artery function.

4. TAKE A BREAK FROM YOUR COMPUTER.
Besides giving you bad posture, being on your computer for extended periods increases your exposure to electromagnetic radiation (EMR). EMR emitting from your computer creates feelings of sluggishness, eye strain, and fatigue. If you work at a computer all day, make sure that you get up and move your body a little at least once an hour, even if it's to walk to the kitchen for a glass of water.

5. CHOOSE ENERGY-BOOSTING SNACKS.
Processed sugar found in foods such as candy and doughnuts creates an instant energy fix but also a dip in energy shortly thereafter. Ditch those sugars in favor of natural snacks that can give your body a boost that will last throughout the day. Nuts are a good choice because they're rich in protein and packed with antioxidants, vitamins, minerals, and omega-3 fatty acids. You can also look for foods with natural sugars and a lower glycemic index, such as berries, which are filled with nutrients and antioxidants that improve mood and promote good digestion.

6. GET 8 HOURS OF SLEEP EACH NIGHT.
Achieving a few rapid eye movement (REM) cycles throughout a full night's sleep has been shown to decrease stress, improve mood, and enhance alertness.

7. HAVE FUN AND LISTEN TO (AND SING) LIVELY MUSIC.

Listening to a favorite song awakens your brain cells and gets your body in sync with a fast-pumping rhythm.

8. EXERCISE IN THE MORNING.

Training in the morning is like waking up your body and preparing it for a day of activity. Inhaling oxygen, challenging your heart, and moving your muscles all promote endurance and energy throughout your day.

9. CONSUME COFFEE MODERATELY.

A cup of joe is not bad for you when you need a big pick-me-up; after all, caffeine increases your memory and alertness. However, too much coffee negatively affects your sleep, stress levels, and blood pressure. Instead, try drinking green tea when you would normally drink coffee during the day. This beverage suppresses your appetite, raises your metabolism, and increases your fat oxidation.

10. HAVE A GOOD LAUGH.

Humor increases vascular blood flow and oxygenation of the blood. As a result you are more alert and creative.

11. USE AROMATHERAPY TO INCREASE ALERTNESS.

Aromatherapy involves sensing and analyzing aromas in the reticular system of the brain stem. Smelling lavender, for example, has calming, relaxing, and balancing benefits.

12. HAVE MORE SEX.

Sex relieves stress, helps you snooze, and increases blood flow in your body.

13. GET OFF SOCIAL MEDIA AND SOCIALIZE IN PERSON.

Socializing has a powerful effect on people's brains and bodies. Being around people improves your mood, posture, and alertness.

14. DRINK MORE WATER.

Water moisturizes your lungs, increases your metabolism, and detoxifies your body.

15. AVOID PEOPLE WHO DRAIN YOUR ENERGY.

Negative people literally "zap" your energy from you. When someone complains or blames constantly, walk quickly in the opposite direction.

HOW TO BUST THE EXCUSE

Write down your schedule and note the times when your energy levels decline. Based on that decline, pick five tips from the list above and start implementing them. Commit to performing them every day for three weeks, and pay close attention to how they impact your energy level.

Excuse #6: I Love Food Too Much

Here's a big secret for those of us who love food: You can be healthy and still eat delicious foods. People who are in great shape also love food. We all love to eat rich, flavorful foods, and we don't want to deny ourselves the pleasure of enjoying a meal. So we don't! It's just that we have figured out a way to make the majority of our meals have the best-quality ingredients.

There is a difference between love and addiction. When you love something, you are able to manage your actions; when you are addicted, you cannot. Ask yourself if you can go a night without dessert, a week without Starbucks, or a month without soda. It's a well-known fact that sugar is addictive, yet it's found in most of our foods. Especially watch out for high fructose corn syrup (HFCS); it's found in nearly everything you eat, from breads, sauces, and juices to cereals and breakfast bars. Think about those favorite foods that you absolutely "love," and you will most likely find this potent and addictive ingredient.

When I was overweight, I thought I loved food. It made me happy when I was sad, distracted me when I was depressed, and calmed me when I had anxiety. I was an emotional eater, a binge eater whose brain didn't register when enough was enough! Asking me to give up cereal, ice cream, and chocolate would be like losing a close friend who had been with me through my hardest life trials.

But I realized that I wasn't eating because I loved food; I was eating because I didn't love myself. I would plow through a bag of chips or a box of cereal without really thinking about it because I wanted to forget whatever was going on in my life. I was in a "zombie eating routine." Break this cycle by noticing when you find yourself eating large quantities even when you're no longer hungry. For me, it's usually when I'm in front of the computer or watching television late at night.

When I realized this unhealthy pattern, I ensured I didn't have those trigger snack foods at my house, and I made a conscious effort not to grab foods when I was bored, distracted, or busy. At one point in my fitness journey I taped the phrase "Nothing Tastes Better Than Being Fit" on my wall to remind me that being healthy was a choice. I needed the reminder of how much happier I would be to feel confident about my health than if I succumbed to another craving. It's not that I was living in a perpetually hungry state; it was about being aware of the difference between a craving and actual hunger. Ultimately, my love for myself became stronger than my love for food.

So, if you find yourself eating without thinking, stop, put the food down, and find a quick distraction. For instance, I have taken the food, thrown it in the trash (making sure it was surely inedible), and then called a friend, gone for a walk, or focused on a creative project. It isn't easy to find a substitute that offers the same instant satisfaction as that snack, but in the process of overcoming your food addiction, you will find discipline, determination, and drive. So it's okay to love food. Just love your health more.

HOW TO BUST THE EXCUSE

Start by being more mindful of your eating habits. How often are you eating because you are hungry, versus eating because there is food in front of you? Loving food means that you should actively enjoy every bite that you take. Do not change your diet drastically in the beginning; just cut your consumption in half. For example, instead of eating a full cheeseburger, just eat half. Chew slowly, enjoy each mouthful, and think about how you feel after each bite. You'll be surprised at what a difference it makes!

Keep in mind that this program doesn't require you to eat 100 percent perfectly. There is no such thing as perfection! I believe in moderation, which is why I follow the 30/30/30/10 program, in which you eat a balanced daily intake of protein, carbohydrates, and fats and if you want, you can utilize that last 10 percent for a small treat!

Create healthier substitutions for the foods you love. If you like eating cheeseburgers, find a healthy alternative, like a turkey burger on a wheat bun with low-fat cheese and minimal sauce. As you rise in your fitness goals you can alter your diet to serve your current purpose, perhaps even removing half the bun or exchanging it for a lettuce wrap. Your new lifestyle isn't about limiting the foods you love; it's about re-creating the foods you love and enjoying the "real thing" once in a while, not every other day.

Excuse #7: I Don't Have Good Genetics

Genetics always plays a small role in your body's physical makeup, but you can combat your susceptibility toward being overweight by eating well and exercising. Everyone faces physical, social, economical, and biological challenges, but you cannot combat them if you compare yourself with unlike individuals. Everyone's body develops differently; some people have a stocky frame while others are a taller, thinner body type. We are all unique, so celebrate the strengths in your genetics instead of focusing on the weaknesses.

Perhaps you have strong shoulders for swimming or muscular calves for running. Don't feel frustrated if you weren't built like a ballet dancer. Your body type may be built for another activity, so it's up to you to discover it! Do the best you can with the cards you were dealt, and don't let them be a self-fulfilling prophecy.

My mother is overweight, and I was always the heaviest of her three daughters. Realizing that my mother's genetics made me susceptible to being overweight prompted me to eat healthy and exercise at a young age. Is it fair that my youngest sister can eat fries, drink wine, and snack on sugar all day and not gain weight? Of course not! But just because it's easier for her doesn't mean I can't have a body I love.

Recognizing your genetic propensity to be overweight should motivate you to work harder. Always remember that while the road ahead is hard, the reward is great. I know that my body is naturally inclined to process food and store fat in a certain way, but I also know I can override that by being smart and strategic. You can, too!

Seek out those who represent your body type and use them as your marker, your basis for comparison.

If you are undergoing any medical treatment, understand that your health situation can be a setback for a while. The most important thing is for you to care for your health and manage your ailment with the help of your doctor. Whatever you are experiencing, keep in mind that a healthy diet and regular physical activity positively benefit the body. Thyroid conditions, for example, are a common medical reason people can't lose weight. While that's a very real obstacle, you need to be vigilant about fixing the problem. Never assume you are overweight because you have an undiagnosed medical condition; get tested before you come to such a conclusion! If you are diagnosed with an underactive thyroid, work with your physician to get it under control.

Or maybe you're dealing with an injury. Don't put undue stress on your body by continuing high-impact exercise. Instead, focus on rest and rehabilitation, because if you are too eager to start training again, it will take longer to heal and you may possibly reinjure yourself. Work around your injury and find exercises that will strengthen your weaknesses and challenge your strengths.

A common ailment preventing people from exercise is fibromyalgia, which is characterized by widespread pain throughout the body, causing stiffness and aches. For many people suffering from this condition, it is hard to move, let alone exercise. However, professionals have strongly recommended exercise as part of a patient's therapy. Encouraging circulation, challenging the heart, and strengthening the muscles is great therapy for any person.

Pregnancy is another medical reason many women don't exercise. While there are certain conditions that require bed rest, most women, especially those who were active before pregnancy, can continue some active fitness program. Generally you don't want your heart rate to go above 140 beats per minute, and as your belly grows, you avoid exercises that require lying on your back. If you sustain an active program and eat 300 to 500 extra calories per day, you can have a healthy pregnancy and even increase your chances for an easier labor.

I have a good friend, Kris Dim, who is a celebrated male body-builder. In the past decade he's undergone three open-heart surgeries and is now paralyzed from the waist down because of a spinal cord injury. Despite his setbacks, on any given morning you will find him at the gym, overcoming his pain and physical limitations by performing upper body exercises, stretching his back, and rehabilitating his legs. So, if you can't run, then swim. If you have injured your knees, train your upper body. If you are sore, focus on stretching. No More Excuses.

When you have physical setbacks, don't use this challenging period to eat unhealthy foods and watch TV. If your activity levels have to decline, focus on what you consume and have your caloric input match your caloric output.

HOW TO BUST THE EXCUSE

Look into your family's medical history and seek areas that will be a struggle for you. Do high blood pressure, high cholesterol, or high blood sugar levels run in your family? Has anyone experienced heart attacks, strokes, or cancer? These are great questions to reflect on now because you can start focusing on prevention.

For instance, if you think you may have a medical condition, get your blood work done promptly to ensure you are properly diagnosed. Follow your doctor's orders while doing what you can to continue challenging your heart and strengthening your muscles. If you are injured, find alternative ways to get your blood flowing without straining yourself. While your exercise level is lower, adjust your caloric and macronutrient intake to reflect your lower activity levels.

No matter what condition your body is in now, there are ways to challenge yourself without risking injury. When I had a sprained ankle, I found that I could use foot straps on my stationary bike to ensure I never applied pressure to the ankle. When I hurt my wrist, I utilized a straight barbell to keep my wrist and forearm in a neutral position as I performed push-ups. When my shoulder blade was inflamed, I avoided running and opted for lighter impact cardio and used the elliptical.

There are many ways to avoid an injury by performing various exercises. For example, you can engage in lower impact exercises like swimming, walking, Pilates, and yoga. Find out if your doctor has any recommendations, listen to your body, and do some research into safe ways to stay active. Pick one activity and commit to it for one full week. Then, reflect on how you feel; if it feels you're making progress, stick with it! If not, pick a different activity and try again.

Excuse #8: I Lack Motivation

It's easier to push yourself to exercise hard and eat right when you have a short-term goal. A lot of people are able to whip their bodies into great shape for a big event, but once the event passes, they resume their old routine of eating poorly and rarely exercising. But this leads to yo-yo dieting that erases results and leaves you feeling frustrated and discouraged. Being fit is a *lifetime* achievement—it can't be just about fitting into a certain size for a specific event. At the end of the day, despite all your excuses, you either want it or you don't. Plain and simple. If you're complacent in your daily routine or overwhelmed with personal and emotional issues, then taking action is really hard. In order to grow, though, you must be challenged—there is no other way. And your challenges must be long term, not just some upcoming deadline.

So challenge yourself and commit to something that scares you. People fail at fitness goals for so many reasons. They fail because there is no sense of urgency, because they don't have the right mind-set, but most of all, because they don't want to succeed.

Yes. I just said that.

People fail because they are too comfortable in their identity. They have written their life story and are comfortable with their current narrative. If you keep saying you're unmotivated because you're tired, depressed, busy, or stressed, then you will seek things in your world to support your claims.

If you want to create motivation, then you must fight the urge to be mediocre and create enough mental discomfort to promote change. Imagine performing a bicep curl with a 5-pound weight. Your muscle isn't challenged because the weight isn't that heavy. Your mind isn't engaged because the challenge isn't great enough. That poor muscle isn't growing because there is not enough opposition. Adversity strengthens you, not weakens you. If you want to create big changes in your body and your life, you need to make yourself *uncomfortable*. You need to feel pressure to change, to keep yourself focused on achieving your goals, regardless of what else is going on in your life. You need to create a mental discomfort zone that will push you out of complacency and force you to grow.

So imagine your best body. Think about how you want to feel, what you want to do, and where you want to go. Envision yourself confidently shopping for sleeveless tops or a form-fitting dress. Picture yourself walking down a beach, hiking up a mountain, or running a 10K race. *Really think about it.* Fill your mind with thoughts of how life would feel if you accomplished this incredible effort to build your best body.

Once you seed a desire, that intention will grow daily through attention, reflection, and action. Put aside some time each week to dream, and allow your thoughts to implant such things in your will.

Think deeply about what achieving your best body really

means. Why do you want it? Choose a deadline and plan a reward when you complete your weight-loss goal. Tell your friends about your efforts and invest in this process. Make yourself accountable to yourself, to your loved ones, to anybody who will keep you going.

When you decide to create a new habit, know that it takes three days to overcome the initial struggle of making it part of your routine. When you pass the three-week mark, you are well on your way to making that change an established habit. By three months, you have ingrained that new habit!

Habits are actions, and actions are what define who we are. And who we are is what we continuously do. When we perform something continuously, it becomes ingrained in the person we are, which alleviates the struggle in trying to find the daily motivation to complete that task. When you develop healthy habits, they are your new standard and no longer a struggle.

Staying motivated in this No More Excuses journey is one of the key ways to ensure your success, so don't take this excuse lightly. Be prepared with a list of things to do when the lack-of-motivation bug bites you. Here are twelve ways to stay motivated:

1. **Enter a competition, either something official or among your friends.**
2. **Plaster motivational quotes all over your house, including your phone's screen saver!**
3. **Post your most inspiring "before" picture on your refrigerator.**
4. **Buy a nice outfit that will fit you in two months and donate your fat clothes.**
5. **Hang around healthy people who motivate you.**
6. **Buy new athletic shoes or a workout outfit.**
7. **Take a group exercise class, try a new workout, or train at a different time of day.**

8. Plan a vacation where you have to wear a swimsuit.

9. Place your alarm clock across your bedroom so that you have to get up to turn it off in the morning.

10. Alarm your cellphone to give you daily reminders to eat, work out, and give gratitude.

11. Volunteer your time with people who don't have full function of their bodies.

12. Buy workout devices like fitness phone applications, a heart rate monitor, or a pedometer.

HOW TO BUST THE EXCUSE

Create a list of personal things that are motivating you to take this fitness journey. Write down twenty-five reasons you want to change your body and your life, even if some of them seem silly, vain, or unimportant. Writing down the reasons you want to make a change to your life will make those reasons feel more real, and looking frequently at the list of reasons will help you stay focused. Remember: good health is the best gift you can give yourself—and you deserve it!

Excuse #9: I Don't Know Where to Start

If you don't know where to start, begin by doing something small. It's as simple as walking 20 minutes this evening or adding a big serving of vegetables to your next meal. Dieting and fitness information can be overwhelming (I know!), and while it's tough to figure out what works, your power is in discovering what works for you! Not everyone can eat a chicken breast and broccoli for lunch five times a week; not everyone likes eating poultry. Not everyone can train with heavy-strength machines because not everyone has access to that equipment. We all have unique allergies, tastes, resources, and physical strengths, so it's up to each of us to figure out where to start.

People often think that a new diet and exercise plan starts in the New Year, on a Monday, or even in the morning. Here's some big news for all of you: You can start right now! You can begin your journey to a healthier you at 3 PM on a Thursday afternoon. The moment you get motivated to change, the minute you unhappily see your reflection in the mirror, and the instant you recognize your dream for a healthy body are the times you need to start taking action! Don't let the moment pass you by; take advantage of that desire and discomfort, and utilize it to create change.

These first few days are exciting times. Not only will you dream big but you will also believe in the power of possibilities. This momentum is what seeds the passion that will elevate you on a journey that will have its peaks and valleys. When you want to give up, this moment is what you will remember best. You can't lose hope; when you're frustrated and tired, you will look back on this moment when you had the most hope—which is right now.

Procrastination and complacency are two big excuses people give for not changing. Many put off what is important for *tomorrow* because of short-term stresses or momentary satisfactions. Maybe you don't feel your weight and unhealthy habits are taking a toll, but it's not a matter of *if*; it's *when*—when your organs, bones, and overall body succumb to the additional pressure you are applying to them. Maybe you won't be able to run with your children, to watch them grow old, or to travel the world in your later years. But if you want a toned body, if you want to see your focus and energy soar, if you want a more healthful life, what on earth are you waiting for?

Every dream begins with a desire. Once that desire takes hold of your psyche, this is the moment to move. Don't wait for tomorrow, don't wait until next week—you need to start now. When you make that decision to change, it has to be a solid thought, stemming from an urgent place.

This book is not about perfection or about beating yourself up if you aren't getting results as quickly as you'd like. *It's about making progress.* It's about not giving up. It's about letting go of guilt or fear of failure and clearing a path for yourself so that success is the easiest option. It's about believing that you deserve to love your body and proving to yourself that you can do *anything* you set your mind to. I will be honest with you: I ate a couple cookies earlier tonight. I was premenstrual, incredibly stressed from work, and fatigued from days on end with the kids. Do I feel bad about it? No. Will I begin anew tomorrow? For sure.

HOW TO BUST THE EXCUSE

The tools and ideas in this book should give you plenty of ways to get started. Since most of our lives are spent lying in bed or sitting in the car, at work, or watching television, it's vital you find opportunities for activity wherever you can. I have been known to walk up and down stairs at airports, perform push-ups at the park, and do lunges while watching television. Here are ten easy ways to incorporate more physical activity into your daily life:

1. **Choose a parking spot that's farther away from your destination.**
2. **Use the stairs instead of the elevator.**
3. **Sit upright when sitting in a chair.**
4. **Perform exercises during commercial breaks on TV.**
5. **Perform push-ups and squats immediately when you rise in the morning.**
6. **Go for an evening walk after dinner.**
7. **Dance along to a fun song (alone or with your kids).**
8. **Take squat breaks every hour.**

9. Stand instead of sit. (I often stand while working, on the phone, and eating.)

10. Stretch while you stand.

Success is not about making huge promises to yourself that will be hard to keep; you will get the results you want by making manageable commitments to yourself and following through—no matter what.

MASTERING YOUR S.T.R.I.V.E.

Bruce Lee wisely said, "Do not pray for an easy life, pray for the strength to endure a difficult one." At this point in our No More Excuses journey, we know that it has not been an easy one. On this road less traveled, many have lacked support, resources, finances, and, oftentimes, faith in this process. As we continue to master our S.T.R.I.V.E. principles, let us remember that stress can work for or against us. How we perceive our circumstances and how we adapt to change will determine our overall success.

In this chapter we will take a good look at our journey so far and begin tackling life—not just fitness—but life. We can't be successful on one end of our life while several other parts deteriorate. We must learn to balance, organize, prioritize, and focus on what's important.

SOME PLATEAU-BUSTING TIPS

If you want to see change, you need to try something different and shock your body! Choose one or two of the following suggestions and incorporate them into your exercise and diet routine.

1. Choose a different cardio exercise.

2. Try new strength exercises.

3. Change the duration of your workout.

4. Switch your intensity level.

5. Lift heavier weights.

6. Increase your repetitions.

7. Raise or lower your caloric intake.

8. Manipulate your macronutrients (i.e., eating lower carbs/higher fats on some days).

9. Invent a new meal plan.

10. Add training days.

Focus on Progress, Not Perfection

Let's get real. You're going to miss workouts. You're going to have an unplanned splurge. You're going to be imperfect in this process because the fact is, nobody is perfect. Not me, not your favorite athlete, and not you. Be forgiving of your weaknesses and focus on your progress. We can always get a little better, and that's the beauty of this journey. Remember that imperfection is perfect. When you strive to attain a higher level of excellence, you are working toward progress. Will you ever reach perfection? No. But the striving to attain it is rewarding in itself and will bring you closer to becoming the person you were meant to become.

The only way to grow is to be challenged. There is no other way. Like the chest muscles that ache while you're pushing through a push-up or adversity in your life that's challenging your mind and spirit, you will become stronger through the process of surviving the pain. So ask yourself: Are you uncomfortable yet? Do your muscles feel sore? Are you pushing yourself hard enough to get results that you're excited about?

If not, let's take a look at some of the things that could be slowing you down. This is a diagnostic test you must regularly run on yourself to ensure you are getting the mileage you want from the vehicle that is your body. If you discover inefficiencies, troubleshoot them. There is no stopping on this road; you are driving and striving to become your very best!

MASTERING THE MACHINE

I often compare the body and its metabolism to a car and its engine. You can't expect your car to perform well if there are inconsistencies in its care. Are you fueling it regularly? Are you getting oil changes and tune-ups? Are you driving it too hard? Are you not driving it at all?

For your body to become a "lean, mean, fat-burning machine," you need to remember the first lesson for success: *consistency*. You must create a trusting environment for you and your body to exist, breed, and progress in. You need to eat at the same time, sleep at the same time for the same length, and poop at the same time—every single day. Your body is a machine, after all, and by giving it proper training, conditioning, and consistency, you can become its effective operator. Most people fail to eat regularly, plateau in their program, suffer from digestive issues, are stressed, and are sleep deprived. If you can master these five elements, you can improve your physical progress and overall quality of life.

PUSH BEYOND THE PLATEAU

If you're being consistent in your plan, whatever was difficult a month ago should now be easier to perform. Perhaps running a mile was difficult at first, but now it's not as much of a challenge. Maybe reducing your calories to a certain number resulted in weight loss initially, but lately you've noticed that you're not getting any slimmer. Your body is always adapting to the pressure, which makes losing weight a double-edged sword. Hitting plateaus is naturally part of this process, and that's actually a good thing: It means that your past efforts have worked!

Remember, though, that challenges are what make you stronger, so you need to create new challenges to continue getting stronger. If you notice your endurance and strength increasing, you should celebrate the fact that your hard work is paying off. Take a week to enjoy and reflect on how far you've come, then think about how you can switch up your exercise program to take yourself to the next level.

If you want to keep building your best body, you're going to have to step up your intensity or change your strategy. To change, you have to challenge yourself more. Sometimes you will spend weeks without seeing any results. Be patient as you persist at this plateau. Continue working hard, staying focused, adjusting your plan, and remaining faithful to your program.

Striving stems from a desire and passion to be better than who you are today. That's why you picked up this book, right? You want to overcome excuses. You want to realize the person you know (and I know) you can become. You have to believe in your power and your purpose. When you start to see your body change, when you start strengthening your mind and empowering your spirit, you will be astounded by the amount of might that you hold within you right now.

LET'S TALK ABOUT FOOD

If you've built a heavy vehicle, that means you've been fueling it with more than it needs to run. But you can't just stop fueling the machine entirely. Most people make the mistake of reducing their fuel intake so much that the engine starts to break down. If you're not fueling your machine, how can you operate? When you are constantly running on empty, it's only a matter of time before your engine starts to stall. Instead, you need to reduce the fuel slowly to ensure you can still operate while improving your body's physical exterior and ultimate performance.

So eat. You should be eating what you usually eat, but a little less each week. Keep in mind that I said a *little*. I didn't say to drop your caloric intake to 1,200 calories a day if you've been consuming 3,000. In fact, if you're hitting a weight-loss plateau right now, it could be because you were overambitious in dropping your caloric intake too early in your program. If you are not eating enough, your body doesn't know what's happening—it thinks there's possibly a famine. So your body begins to store fat and burn calories at a slower rate.

You are doing a disservice to your diet if you're dieting too much. If you aren't feeding your body enough, your body will reduce the speed it takes to process foods, so it can burn at the new pace you are feeding it. Your body is an adaptable machine and will adjust itself according to the stimuli placed upon it. So start eating more regularly and increase your calories if you're not giving your body enough nutrients. The goal isn't to eat the *least* amount of food; the goal is to master your metabolism and have it serve you.

HELLO, JOHN!

If you are eating, then you should be digesting. There is no set rule for how often you should be "on the john," but you should be urinating every one to two hours and have a bowel movement every one to two days. Unfortunately, Americans struggle with this single "act," with the laxative industry making $725 million annually.

The perfect bowel movement is experienced without difficulty and the stool floats (at first). How does it smell? Does it stick to the toilet bowl? Are you straining? Is your toilet time a 10-minute event? These are great questions you can ask yourself as you are becoming the master of your machine. There is no better sign of good health than how your body processes foods.

When I'm not regular, I know something is wrong. I'm either eating unhealthy foods, I'm too stressed, or I'm not drinking at least eight 8-ounce glasses of water a day. Nothing is more evident of that than after a huge splurge day, when I'm literally hunched over on the john somewhere, wishing I had had more discipline the day before. It's not just the frequency you should consider, it's also the size and shape that should concern you.

FIVE WAYS TO IMPROVE YOUR DIGESTION

1. *Find your body's rhythm:* Seek the time of day your body likes to excrete.

2. *Go raw:* Consume three servings of raw fruits and vegetables daily.

3. *Drink vinegar:* Consume 1 to 3 teaspoons of apple cider vinegar alongside some water and perhaps honey (if needed); you can take them before meals or once daily using a straw.

4. *Get moving:* Encourage blood circulation through daily movement.

5. *Start meditating:* Relax your body and prepare it to release.

I discovered I can't eat a lot of sugar, drink milk, or consume artificial sweeteners—based on my output. In limiting them in my diet, not only did my digestive system become more efficient but I also began to effectively lose weight.

LOWER YOUR STRESS LEVEL

Stress can kill. I'm sure you've heard that before, but I can't emphasize enough how bad stress truly is. Not only can stress make you hold on to toxins in your body, but it can also indirectly cause heart disease, high blood pressure, and chest pain. If not managed well, you will find yourself struggling with all kinds of related issues, from mindless eating to impulsive anger, to living a poor quality of life.

When you're stressed, your body creates a "fight or flight" response, in which adrenaline and cortisol are released. The hormone cortisol—a.k.a. the stress hormone—increases your insulin production, making you hungry, as well as promotes the accumulation of belly fat. You need to find a strategy for combating the specific stresses you're under, and that strategy has to be one you can realistically practice on a regular basis. Sure, a weekend getaway at a nice spa will reduce your stress level, but who can pull that off all the time?

If you see your weight-loss results slowing down, and you've taken a good look at your eating habits, the next thing to check is your stress-management habits. Try something new; some people exercise, go for a walk, focus on breathing, talk to a friend, write, pray, meditate, or listen to music. For some people, just enjoying a cup of tea can be enough. I work out when I am stressed. Stress is a strong energy that needs to be released in the form of a positive action; if I can't exercise, I go for a walk. If I can't walk, I write. If I can't write, I call someone. If there is no one to call, I get on my knees and start praying!

Dieting can stress you out, especially if you start getting frustrated by the program. Believe me, I get it! But remember, this No More Excuses program is not about being perfect—it's about discovering who you are and bettering yourself every day through triumphs *and* failures. I want you to push yourself on this program, but I also need you to believe that YOU CAN DO THIS. There is no obstacle that we cannot overcome together.

Don't let negative energy breed and build inside of you. You must transform and transfer it to another place, because here's a secret: When you're in control of it, stress makes you stronger. For instance, when you strategically apply stress when running, it makes your heart stronger. When you deliberately impose stress on your muscles by squatting, your legs become stronger. When you are running a household, working and raising children, that stress can make you more focused and effective.

So take a step back and make a plan for how to take control of the stressors in your life. Use the S.P.E.E.D. model. Give yourself a quick break to get focused and organized, and you will become a better version of yourself and those you serve, including your family, friends, employers, and community.

TIME YOUR TASKS

Everyone has the same 24 hours in a day. If you find yourself limited in time and failing to finish your to-do list daily, then you need to examine where you can make more time. While there can be a multitude of tasks that fill a day, the truth is that some people use their time better than others. Some people wake up with a goal in mind and know exactly how they will achieve it. They prepared for the day in advance. They visualized how they will perform each action to reach that goal. They have a positive mind-set with preparations in case things go wrong.

You will be amazed at how you are able to find the time to achieve your goals when you have them clearly in mind! If you understand why you want to complete something, the how of doing it becomes very easy. You will make it happen if it is truly important to you. For instance, if you knew that exercising today would help you lose 8 pounds this month, and ultimately 50 pounds in the next six months, then you would be a lot more likely to succeed than if you had only a vague idea that working out will help you look better in the long run.

WAKE UP WITH GOALS IN MIND

There will always be routine things, like cleaning, cooking, studying, working, and managing a household, that you will *have* to do. So how do you make time for yourself? First, remember that taking care of your health is something that you're doing for everybody; it's not just for vanity, it's not a luxury—it's an absolute necessity if you want to live a long and enjoyable life. Here are some other tips for finding extra time:

1. WAKE UP EARLIER.

After getting a minimum of 7 hours of sleep, schedule your wake-up to be 30 to 60 minutes before you have to actually start your day. The very best time to work out is in the morning. You get it done before you have time to talk yourself out of it! You can follow a DVD in your pajamas at home or sleep in your training clothes and head to the gym.

2. CUT OUT TV WATCHING.

The average American watches 34 hours of TV a week. That's 4 to 5 hours per day! Many stay-at-home moms rely on daily talk shows to stay connected to the outside world; working folks use television to "zone out" after a stressful day. We watch our favorite reality, singing, and drama shows to give ourselves a mental break, which is understandable. Here's the thing, though: Not only does television make you more tired but it also wastes so much of your life. The amount of time you spend watching TV can be applied to time with family and friends, going for a walk, getting organized, cooking, working out, or doing something productive that moves you toward reaching your goals.

THREE-DAY TV DETOX

If your TV time is the only break you give yourself, you need to try this today! For the next three days, skip your shows. Use the entire time that you would be watching TV to work on your S.P.E.E.D. goal—planning meals, preparing food, or working out. If you finish your tasks before the end of your TV time, sit on the floor in your TV room, turn on some relaxing music, and work on your flexibility. Use the exercises in this book to stretch, flex, and open up your body. If you usually watch TV by yourself, don't let anybody interrupt you—this is your time! If you have a TV buddy, invite the person to join you!

3. LIMIT YOUR INTERNET BROWSING.

The latest study shows that the average person spends 8 hours a week on Facebook. OMG! Right there are all the hours you need to work out! I know it's a hard sell to give up Internet browsing (even for me), but you *can* browse differently. Most of the time I can check Facebook while waiting in the grocery line or while on a StairMaster (making sure I'm still at my target heart rate, of course). There's nothing wrong with a little online socializing, but discipline yourself to do it after you've completed your daily tasks. If it doesn't help you toward your long-term goals, it is hurting you.

4. SQUEEZE IN WORKOUTS WHENEVER YOU CAN.

Quality workouts are defined by intensity and focus rather than duration. If you can get your heart churning and muscles pumping in a 30-minute time frame, then you've got it made! Make the time to work out by incorporating fitness whenever you can fit it in; this may be during your lunch break or on your way home after work. You can train while watching your kids play at the park or while the baby is napping. I have jumped rope and performed burpees while supervising my sons in the backyard! Commit to getting your exercise in no matter what, and suddenly you will start seeing opportunities everywhere.

5. SCHEDULE EXERCISE INTO YOUR CALENDAR.

If you live by a long to-do list, make sure that your health is front and center on it! If you jot it down, it becomes a goal that you get to check off when it's done, before moving to the next thing. You don't want it to be the task that you do after all of your "real" responsibilities and obligations are fulfilled. I hate to break it to you, but the to-do list is never going away; you will always have one more task or one more item that you could be taking care of before you make time for yourself. So, when you create your daily schedule, include time to work out, just as you would schedule a meeting or an appointment.

6. GO TO SLEEP!

Don't ever underestimate the power of a good night's sleep. Not only will it make you alert and refreshed, but it will also help you lose weight! Yes, even resting helps you lose weight. If you don't sleep well, that can alter your hormones and increase your appetite. Aim for a minimum of 7 hours of sleep each night.

If you are having a tough time sleeping, here are some suggestions:

- ☐ **STOP EATING CLOSE TO BEDTIME.**

- ☐ **START A NIGHTTIME ROUTINE.**

- ☐ **SAY A PRAYER OR MEDITATE BEFORE BEDTIME.**

PRAYERS AND MEDITATIONS

Before you sleep, reflect on your day and think about what you're grateful for. When you focus on things you have, versus what you don't have, you create spiritual abundance in your life. By thinking of the positive, you see events, people, and things in a new light. Much of what happens around us is out of our control, but if we can control how we react to any situation, good or bad, we gain power beyond measure. Before bedtime, say:

Today I am grateful for. . .

Thank you for. . .

Help me with. . .

. . . so I can become the best version of myself.

Some Principles and Some Examples

You are the master of your universe. When you produce an action, it creates an outcome. This is a simple law of cause-and-effect. I didn't make this up; this is a universal principle. If you water a seed, it will grow. If it doesn't grow, give it some sunlight. If it doesn't thrive, change the soil. Whatever you do, keep taking action because eventually you will master the process.

The most powerful part of this law is realizing that the person who is behind any action is you. If you can master your mind, then you can control your actions. If you can control your actions, then you can dictate your future. Nothing is more evident of this principle than when you are building your best body. Be prepared to dream big, work hard, and constantly reflect.

If you think failure isn't part of this process, think again. We have all failed at one point or another. For example, I failed when I gained 30 pounds from eating my emotions for more than three years. I failed when I put myself last on my priority list of the day. I failed when I ate healthy through an entire family event, only to come home and binge on ice cream, chocolate, and chips. I have definitely failed countless times in my life, but I have never given up. When I woke up, I dwelled on my past actions, but didn't allow them to define me.

LET GO OF THE PAST

It's not worth thinking about the workout you missed or the craving you caved in to the day before. The past is past. It's done! It's over with. There is absolutely nothing you can do to change the action you performed last week, yesterday, or 5 minutes ago. Thinking about it, stressing over it, being depressed because of it will not change it. How powerful is that?

The only thing regrets do is settle into your soul and make you feel shame. Yet there is nothing shameful about the struggle. No one is perfect, which is why the person who gets to the finish line quicker is the one who later fails the fastest. Following the S.P.E.E.D. method by Setting, Planning, Envisioning, Executing, and Delivering a result doesn't *guarantee* your desired result; it means it creates *some* result. If that result isn't what you want, then you need to change your plan. For example, if you find that your strict diet and ambitious workout plan are falling short weekly, then adjust your goals to make them attainable and achievable. If you notice a place, person, or thing that doesn't promote your healthy plan, then make adjustments in your future interactions. Being fluid and amenable to change is an important aspect of your success.

Let's consider an example. Shelly Newby has always been an athlete. In high school, she could jump the highest, run the fastest, hit the hardest, and score the most—she once had 36 points in a basketball game. In college, she became a model, displaying her svelte physique. When she had children, she stopped exercising and devoted her attention to raising kids. In the past five years, she has become a single mom, turned 36, and decided to begin focusing on her health.

Unfortunately, during this time she also received bad news from her doctor. She underwent surgery for both thyroid and breast cancer. When she thought the fight was over, another doctor diagnosed her with Hashimoto's and multiple sclerosis, both auto-immune diseases. She finally stopped living in the success of her past and declared war on her ailments. She needed to fight for her health and become a positive presence for her children. After reading constant studies on the importance of movement and disease prevention, she joined a gym after a ten-year absence.

When Shelly started, she felt overweight, intimidated, overwhelmed, and insecure. Most of all, she felt ashamed and embarrassed that she had "let herself go." Though she lacked time and motivation, she clocked in at 5 AM at the gym before she headed to work each day. While her results are slower due to her thyroid medications, she isn't giving up. She has lost 18 pounds in 6 months and gone from a size 14 to a size 10. Now Shelly has more energy and proudly hikes with her kids.

ADAPTATION IS THE CRUX OF YOUR STRENGTH AND ENDURANCE

Your mind, body, and spirit will be challenged by the continuous changes you're applying to your new lifestyle. Most actions are habits. What you're trying to create is a new set of healthy habits that will lead you to a desired, healthier outcome. The changes involved in this effort are not easy; they require you to make deliberate choices every day that call for continuous thought. The strain in mentally disciplining your actions and physically pushing your body's limits will not be easy, but if you can move with the challenges and adjust to the changes, you can progress in your efforts.

Maybe waking up an hour earlier is tough. Perhaps incorporating more protein into your meals is not easy. Oftentimes, things don't go as planned; children get sick and all of a sudden avoiding your favorite dessert or a cold can of beer can be difficult. However, if you can meet these challenges by adapting your solutions, substituting your favorite meals, and staying focused on your long-term goals, you can win this No More Excuses game.

Keep in mind that your program can be changed at any time. If you notice you clock in only 3 miles a week, thereby failing your 10-mile weekly goal, change that goal to 5 miles until you master that distance. Adapt and adjust according to your challenge. Change, whether good or bad, is hard for anyone to deal with, but the faster you adapt to these changes, the sooner you can see your success.

SUCCESS IS AN ACCUMULATION OF SMALL VICTORIES

Losing weight is not only a science but also a math equation. If your goal is to lose 50 pounds, focus on losing 10 pounds five times. If your goal is to run a 5K race, run an extra 2 kilometers every couple weeks until you meet your goal. That is, whenever you set a long-term goal, it is helpful to break down the steps to achieve it, setting a series of intermediate goals. So what is the very first step that will lead you toward the next step? Keep your eye on the achievable prize. If you focus on what you can do, versus what you can't yet do, then you open yourself up to the possibility of achieving that grander goal.

Let's consider another example. At his heaviest, Eli Sapharti weighed nearly 300 pounds. Every day he smoked two packs of cigarettes and drank two liters of soda. In 2008, he had high blood pressure, aching joints, severe anxiety, panic attacks, and constant fatigue. In addition to his physical symptoms, emotionally he was drained and in the process of ending his eighteen-year-long marriage.

One day, he received a wake-up call when a salesclerk told him he was "really good-looking for an overweight guy." That comment and the obese reflection that stared back at him in the mirror made him realize that he did, in fact, look much older than his 38 years. Unlike the quick fixes and fad diets he had unsuccessfully tried in the past, Eli decided to escape his downward spiral and seek long-term results by taking each day one step at a time.

By celebrating his small victories he lost more than 100 pounds, stopped smoking, and replaced his fizzy-drink intake with water. Today, Eli runs, weight-trains, and follows a healthy diet of lean protein, whole grains, vegetables, and other foods in moderation. He is now 180 pounds with 10 percent body fat. He even found love again and is set to marry later this year.

WHEN YOU LEAST WANT TO IS WHEN IT MATTERS MOST

It's easy to perform tasks when you are motivated and inspired, whether it's being on a strict diet, vowing yourself in marriage, or working for a corporation. What really measures your level of commitment is putting in an effort when you have no desire. What do you do when you're on your third day of eating unhealthy and have already missed a week of workouts? How do you do when the scale hasn't budged and you have even gained weight? How do you react when your spouse puts you down or your boss adds more work to your already stress-filled job? What do you do when the last thing you want to do is put on your athletic shoes and work out?

You go work out. You work out even though every fiber of your being is saying "No, don't do it." You do it. You get it done. Even if it's just 20 minutes, you do something progressive that's for you, for your health, and for your self-confidence. Think about those small victories and count your action plan backward, realizing that the small decision to follow through today is what will lead you to the next big victory. Disciplining your mind and forcing it to perform actions it doesn't want to perform is power gained. The ability to zero in on your long-term mission and focus on getting a task done, despite your desire not to, will deepen your resolve and destiny will be determined by you.

FOCUS ON WHAT YOU CAN DO VERSUS WHAT YOU CAN'T

When someone goes on a diet, the first thing that person thinks about is all the things he or she can't do. He can't eat the normal, unhealthy foods he enjoys. She can't sit and watch endless TV. But there can be No More Excuses! Nobody likes restrictions; after all, limitations usually make people want to break them. So don't think about limitations.

Don't think about the foods you can't eat or the things you can't do because you have committed yourself to working out that evening. Think instead about all the foods you can choose from. Think about all the things you can do once you build your strength and endurance. Think about being confident, feeling beautiful, and knowing that you are living an intentional life. You aren't restricted, limited, or constrained—you are consciously choosing the harder route because you desire a bigger reward.

Freedom is the ability to choose your actions and not be limited by food addictions, peer pressure, or an uncomfortable physique. Every day you must remind yourself that this new journey is not something you have to do, it's something you want to do. It's your choice.

COMPLACENCY KILLS, CHALLENGES BUILD

It's much easier to live an involuntary life, during which you wake at the same time, drive the same route, eat the same foods, watch the same shows, and get stressed, depressed, and distressed over life's uncontrollable events. You can either continue what you've always been doing and get what you've been getting, or you can change your routine and achieve a different result. When you live a mediocre existence, you aren't trying—you're not striving, you're just surviving. You're getting by, getting through, and getting old in the process.

If you desire something greater for yourself, then you have to stop the routine. You have to wake up! You have to get uncomfortable because the only way to grow is to become challenged. Once the thought of greatness enters your mind, though, be prepared for a shock. You will discover your favorite coffee drink takes up the majority of your allotted daily calories. You will uncover supposed friends who are unsupportive of your efforts. You will realize pieces of yourself that are weak, fragile, and easily tempted.

Don't feel frustrated by this process. While complacency seemingly feels like the easier route, living an unfulfilled, unhealthy, and unrealized life is much harder. You are much greater than this moment. Ten years from now, you will regret not completing this challenge.

Maria Romey lost 40 pounds in four months after she saw an unflattering picture of herself in a bridesmaid's gown at her friend's wedding. She knew her weight was creeping up, and while her mother made small jabs about her growing size, she didn't care. She was enjoying carefree dinners with friends, drinks with coworkers, and late-night pizzas with her long-term boyfriend. She was comfortable with her lifestyle and complacent about her physical goals—that is, of course, until she saw that picture.

She began taking dance classes and learned how to strength-train. She slowly altered her diet and created supportive friendships. Looking back, she realized that she didn't have an excuse for being overweight. Her "excuse" was that she didn't care about living a healthy lifestyle. She was comfortable with her routine and didn't desire to change because most friends enabled her unhealthy habits. It wasn't until she became critical of her body in that bridesmaid's dress that she felt truly uncomfortable and sought to create change.

NOTHING GREAT COMES WITHOUT SACRIFICE

You will risk a lot in this No More Excuses journey. You will reorganize and prioritize your life. You will apply more effort toward realizing your dreams, and in the process, you will exert more energy in planning healthy meals and making time for exercise. You may lose peers who saw you as the eating-out buddy, the drinking comrade, or the partying pal. You will sacrifice your time, your resources, and your friendships at some point, but know that it won't be forever.

There is an end to your current destination, so if you feel overwhelmed by the sacrifices, know that once you reach your resolution, your program will *change*. You will always strive, but your striving will get easier. It will shift in different directions. Don't feel defeated by the moment; realize that this sacrifice occurs for a positive long-term effect. When you find purpose in your pain, you will feel better about those seemingly hard choices you make today.

PERCEIVE, BELIEVE, ACHIEVE—IT HAPPENS IN THAT ORDER

The first step you take in this No More Excuses journey is to examine your perception. What do you see? What kind of success do you want? Who do you want to become? How long do you want to live? You must *perceive* your success as realizable in order to start believing in it. Once you start believing in yourself and your abilities, this journey will unveil opportunities to make it happen.

You absolutely cannot achieve something if you do not see it and believe it first. If you're feeling doubtful or insecure, then develop that "mental muscle" now. Your mind will fluctuate; sometimes you'll feel defeated, other times you'll feel accomplished; sometimes you'll feel tired, other times you'll feel energetic. Regardless of what peak or valley you're hitting on this journey, you have to always believe in your strength and ability to conquer. Achievement begins and ends with the mind.

I met Alma Gutiérrez at a park during one of my No Excuse Mom meet-ups. She was a nanny of two young boys, and I asked her to join us. Initially she declined, later admitting that she was uncomfortable, insecure, and didn't feel "fit" enough to exercise with us. She soon became a regular attendee, though, writing down her food intake and running daily. This was a big step for her self-esteem because she was always the heavier daughter among her six sisters. For most of her life Alma believed she was genetically inclined to be heavy. When she started believing in her ability to change her physique, though, she began achieving incredible results, losing 30 pounds in just three months.

GIVE LIFE JUST 3 PERCENT MORE EFFORT

How much effort can you make to live this life? Can you hold your plank a little longer? Can you lift a little more? If you perceive all exertion on a scale of 1 to 10, then when you're near the top—at level 9—try to do 3 percent more. That is, can you do three more push-ups, run 3 minutes longer, or do three extra burpees? That little effort—that small percentage added to what you perceive as your top ability—makes you stronger. Three minutes is a commercial break. It's a stoplight! It's a short moment in time when you challenged yourself and invested in a long-term vision.

If you live each day properly challenging yourself so that you're not overexerting your efforts but incrementally adding that 3 percent ability, you can grow without undue strain. In any race, the difference between first and second place is a small percentage; so, too, is the extra effort to be made in pushing beyond a weight-loss plateau. Push yourself, challenge yourself, and amaze yourself by reaching a perceived level of 9 and then going beyond what you believed your body could do.

STRIVING MAKES YOU HAPPY

Have you ever won a contest, participated in a race, taken a vacation, or attended an event, only to feel a little let down at the end? It's common to feel a small bout of depression after a big accomplishment, because all of your mental and physical efforts were used to prepare for that accomplishment and then it's over. While it was engaging, challenging, and frustrating, it was a focused effort that created a desired result, which was rewarding.

When you focus on your strengths, you become at "flow" with your life. Flow is when you are immersed in an activity and your engagement eliminates the time spent. While you are challenged, the effort makes you happy, an observation developed by positive psychologist Mihaly Csikszentmihalyi. Like playing a board game, working out, or cooking meals, the efforts involved when you are active (versus passive, like watching TV) make you feel both lost in and engaged with the process. For instance, you often hear that happiness is in the travel, not in the destination.

Whether you realize it or not now, the discipline, dedication, desire, faith, focus, and effort you put into staying on course make you mentally, physically, and spiritually better. You will uncover your strengths, recognize your weaknesses, work toward realizing your goals, and keep your eye on your prize. The ability to master your mind will unlock endless future goals beyond your current endeavors. The strive to attain self-mastery is making you stronger, happier, and wiser.

PART 4

S.C.O.R.E.

Speculate

Celebrate

Operate

Rejuvenate

Evaluate

YOUR NEW NORMAL

Congratulations! You found ways to S.T.R.I.V.E. to get ahead, even when distractions were thrown in your way. You stayed focused with S.P.E.E.D., and you've worked hard to achieve your goal. It's time to celebrate winning this battle to create your best body! The next chapter will help you do that, and take you even further.

At the same time, however, let's make sure you keep that best body by developing a manageable maintenance plan. It is often said that losing weight is the easy part, but that keeping it off is the hard part. So let's create a plan to keep it off.

The Road Ahead

It's amazing that you are in such a great place right now, but that doesn't mean you will be next week, or next month, or next year. Things will constantly challenge you to maintain your good state of health. There will be stress, children, age, holidays, injuries, and depression; you'll test your ability to eat clean, exercise, and stay focused on fitness. As management guru Dan Rockwell has said, "If you think you've arrived, you aren't where you think you are."

For you to keep growing, you need to keep improving and remain on top of your physical condition. That means you need to continuously challenge yourself. You may be saying, "I'm fine with the way I look." And you should love the way you look, but you have to remember what it took to get you there. Complacency challenges not just your fitness, but also your relationships, your work, and your overall life. You must do what so many have a hard time doing, which is to appreciate what you have, daily. You must cherish, change, and challenge yourself regularly to maintain and increase the things you appreciate in your life.

The number one reason I stay motivated is that I walk a fine line between being satisfied and wanting a little more. In the beginning of my fitness journey, I wanted to lose 15 pounds. After I lost that weight, I wanted to see definition in my abs. Then I wanted to have stronger shoulders, then rounder glutes, and a cleft in my arms. After a while, I wanted to perform 10 pull-ups, run a half-marathon, and dead-lift 150 pounds. Years later, I wanted to lose weight after having children, look great at a holiday event, or be prepared to wear a bikini when I took my sons swimming. I always worked on my goals in twelve-week stages, I always kept a calendar for recording my accountability, and I always centered my life as a mentor, a supporter, and a follower.

A maintenance plan does not necessarily mean that you will continue to "diet" as you have. It also doesn't mean that you will go straight back into eating out, drinking alcohol, and oversplurging on sweet treats. *You can never go back to the way you were.* I repeat: you *cannot* go back to the lifestyle you once had.

You must create a new normal. This new normal will require you to eat healthfully and will allow you to indulge mindfully. This new normal also means you will eat the number of calories you need to sustain the new person you have created.

The Person You Have Become

You must eat like the person you have become. If your caloric intake is 1,600 calories a day at the weight you exist at now, you need to stay near that caloric number to maintain your body. You should continue to follow the 30/30/30/10 macronutrient guide and eat a balanced diet with lean protein, complex carbohydrates, and unsaturated fats; but you can feel free to take that 10 percent and splurge a little or alter a macronutrient depending on your activity levels. In essence, you don't have to be as strict as you were when you were dieting, but you must stay at your new body's caloric target.

This means you can add some carbohydrates after 4 PM, drink some wine, or have a fancy coffee once in a while. And you can enjoy two or three small treat meals during the week, again as long as you stay at your caloric target and continue your exercise regimen. You realize that you are an adult and you choose what you put in your body. Choose the wrong things and you will suffer the consequences of how it will make you feel. When you have cleansed your system, for instance, your body will negatively react to too much sugar, saturated fats, and alcohol. The best diet is a healthy diet, with occasional splurges.

If you've been training three to five days a week and want to cut back, you can certainly cut back a little, but don't cut back a lot. The best way for your body to maintain its current physique is for you to get continuous oxygen from cardiovascular exercise and muscle from strength exercises. To keep your interest, you can try various classes, run at different intensities, and play with your rep ranges and sets. You don't have to work harder; you just have to continuously challenge your body and try different things.

If you don't monitor your food intake or your fitness activity, you can easily go south without knowing it! I recommend continuing your fitness calendar and writing down your food intake until you feel comfortable with your new normal. For the last fifteen years, I've kept a fitness calendar taped to my wall, even after I hit my fitness goals. Keeping the calendar reminded me to stay consistent and to work toward the next goal.

Mistakes You Shouldn't Make

Let's talk about why people sometimes fail in this department and how you can avoid making that mistake yourself.

1. THEY ARE BURNED OUT.

When you change your lifestyle drastically in a twelve-week period, it can really take a toll on your body and mind. Imagine climbing an endless, steep mountain and wanting to rest afterward. If you climbed very fast, without properly fueling or pausing, then your body is literally burned out and you'll be trying to rebuild after all that "torture." For many people, the physical and mental impact of an exercise plan is so great that it halts continued progress and kills any desire to make it up the next summit. This is why making small adjustments to your lifestyle is the best route. You change your habits slowly and acquire the small yet significant strength needed to take on this journey, one step at a time.

2. THEY DON'T SET A NEW GOAL.

Life is endless goal seeking. It's hard to think of life in these infinite terms because we constantly focus on happiness as a destination and not the journey. Why focus on an end result if you know that it will not make you happy, right? The truth is, it *will* make you happy but for only a limited amount of time. Think about a moment you received the newest technology or finished a long-awaited vaca-

tion. It's fun for a bit, but that happiness fades. To constantly progress (and stay happy), you always need a destination ahead, one
that will keep your mind in flow by physically and mentally challenging you.

3. THEY DON'T HAVE A SUCCESSFUL ENVIRONMENT.

Your environment is not just about the gym you train at, the foods
in your cabinet, or the new running shoes in your closet. The most
important aspect of your environment is the people inside it. In the
previous chapter, I talked about your mentor, your supporter, and
your follower. These three people are who will keep you on track
also when you're in maintenance mode. Your mentor will note your
complacency. Your supporter will encourage you to stay focused.
And your follower will look to you for inspiration. There is an invisible pressure to not fail these people. If you are the only person who
trekked uphill, then it's only harder to continue going it alone.

4. THEY DON'T HAVE THE RIGHT MENTALITY.

Every day you have to wake up with feelings of gratitude. It's hard to
be grateful for your now-fit physique because you have it, of course.
It seems we always want what we don't have, but we forget to appreciate what we do have. But the right mentality means appreciating
your health each day. It also means being cognizant of when your
mind turns "lazy" about making healthy choices. For instance, it
can seem that twelve weeks can pass pretty slowly when you're on
the journey, but when it ends you think, "Wow, I'm pretty proud
of myself! If I gain a couple pounds, I now know what to do to lose
the weight!" So you indulge in some cupcakes, happy hours, and
missed workout sessions. Two extra pounds becomes 5 pounds,
5 pounds becomes 10—you get the picture. Before you know it, you
are right back where you were because you thought, "I can lose
weight whenever I want." Don't ever forget how hard the battle was
fought.

5. THEY ARE BIOLOGICALLY CHALLENGED.

Fat cells can shrink but they won't go away. According to a 2008 Swedish study published in the journal *Nature,* the number of fat cells stays constant throughout a person's life. This explains why it's so hard to lose weight and maintain your physique. There are 25 to 30 billion fat cells in a normal person's body (triple in those who are obese), and when you gain weight, the cells just get bigger. If your cells grow extensively, they will split and create more fat cells! When you lose weight, alas, you don't burn fat cells, you just shrink them.

I repeat: You don't burn fat cells, you just shrink them. This means that your body will be fighting to get back to what is "normal" for it (imagine a deflated balloon). Your body is going to want to refill its fat cells and return to its set point weight. Set point weight is a theory that your body, regardless of weight gained or lost, will desire to return to a set point range. As you lose weight, your metabolism slows down because it begins conserving the minimal calories you are now feeding it. Your slower metabolism, coupled with hormonal changes, creates additional challenges in maintaining your new weight loss.

Does this mean you are out of luck? Absolutely not. My set point weight has changed several times throughout the years. In my late teens, my 5-foot-4-inch frame was 115 to 120 pounds. In my mid-twenties, I was 145 to 155 pounds. While pregnant, I was 175 to 180 pounds, and now I've settled at 125 to 130 pounds. I have stayed several years at each of these weight stages. My set point was consistent during those times, and the number of fat cells didn't change. The only things that changed were my eating habits, hormonal challenges, activity expenditure, and, of course, pregnancy.

When I finally reached my current weight, it was a battle to keep it off. After I reached my fitness goal of running a half-marathon, completing a photo shoot, or taking a beach vacation, I regressed a little when I took a full exercise and diet break. I started not watching what I ate, not training as intensely, and not sleeping enough. As soon as I saw my weight climb back up, though, I refocused, lost the weight, and developed a maintenance plan to keep my weight off.

The Maintenance Plan

Creating a successful maintenance plan requires you to continue striving to reach long-term goals. You do this by utilizing the No More Excuses accountability tools, but at this point you can be more flexible in your dieting and exercise. So let's review the steps for developing a maintenance program.

STEP ONE: CREATE A NEW FITNESS CALENDAR

Keep a continuous fitness calendar hanging on your wall. Create it every three months. Write down your new goals and reflect on the months passed. Strive for consistency and see the calendar as a visual reminder to get moving.

STEP TWO: RECALCULATE YOUR CALORIC NEEDS

Return to Chapter 7 and the discussion of caloric needs in weight-loss mode. After your transformation, you will need to recalculate how many calories your body needs for your current weight and activity level. Based on the 30/30/30/10 formula, alter your macronutrients in accordance with your daily activities, and perhaps utilize that last flexible 10 percent to enjoy small splurges. For instance, enjoy a handful of M&M's or a bite of dessert. But stay within your caloric range and maintain your balanced meals throughout the day. Make sure you are inputting the right number of calories for your new caloric output.

STEP THREE: DESIGN A NEW EXERCISE REGIMEN

As you age—and we are all aging—your muscles begin to deteriorate. These small changes start occurring around age 30. You get injured easier, you become less flexible, and you don't heal as quickly. In your forties, people lose an average of 1 to 2 percent of muscle mass per year! If you think maintenance means decreasing your exercise output, though, think again. If you want to keep what you have, you will have to work at it.

If you haven't dabbled enough in strength training during your weight-loss phase, now is the time to start lifting, squatting, curling, and pressing! Design a new exercise regimen that focuses on building and maintaining muscle mass, challenging your heart through cardio training, and ultimately increasing your metabolism. Your maintenance program should include a continuous exercise routine complete with cardio, strength, and flexibility training. Strive for a minimum of three days a week of exercise, and focus on challenging yourself a little more each week.

STEP FOUR: BECOME A ROLE MODEL

You have succeeded at a goal that 70 percent of Americans attempt to reach. You will be celebrated, admired, maybe even scorned, for achieving your weight-loss mission. Identify and position yourself as the fitness friend, the one who's maintained her weight loss and practices healthy habits. When you step out as a healthy role model among your community of family and friends, you will be held to higher expectations. Those social expectations will force and encourage you to stay on course when you want to have a large piece of pie or slack off on your runs. Instead, start giving back, providing tips and becoming a helpful friend to those who are still fixing their life vehicles.

STEP FIVE: SET A NEW GOAL

In Part 3, you learned the S.T.R.I.V.E. principles, and you understand the importance of constantly seeking improvement. This journey to protect, strengthen, and maintain your body won't end until the day you don't need your physical functions anymore. You get the idea. So start your engines and drive to a new destination with S.P.E.E.D.

Set your eyes on new fitness goals. Plan your journey with new exercises and a 30/30/30/10 macronutrient profile that supports those new goals. Envision succeeding and overcoming the new hurdles you will face in the next three months, and then start executing your plan. Once you deliver the results and reflect on a weekly basis, try harder the next week. Don't stop until you S.C.O.R.E.—but that's the next chapter!

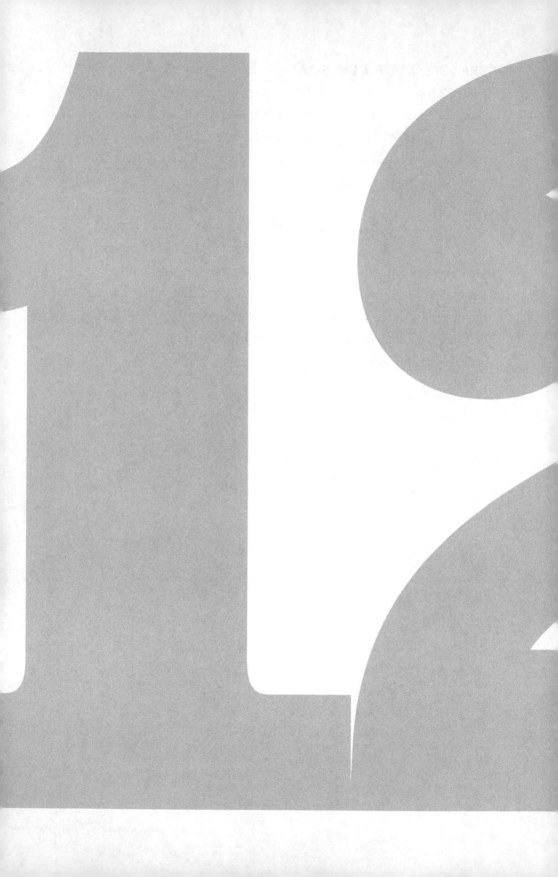

S.C.O.R.E. AND KEEP MOVING

S.C.O.R.E.! You've made it. You've reached your short-term goal! You've lost weight, gained muscle, increased your endurance, enhanced your strength, and improved your flexibility. Not only have you built your confidence, but you have also mastered the ability to set goals, plan a strategy, envision success, execute day after day, and deliver results. Congratulations! Relish your success and reflect on your No More Excuses journey. While you may not be exactly where you want to be yet, you need to take a break from the hustle and celebrate how far you've come.

I can still distinctly remember the celebratory moments when I achieved a goal, whether it was competing on stage, fitting into my post-pregnancy jeans, or confidently wearing a bikini at the beach. Working in three-month increments reminded me always that there was an end to every effort and that I could rest once I achieved my goals before beginning the next stretch. Your body, mind, and spirit have worked harder, trained harder, and pushed harder than ever before. Now it's time for a bit of rest. Your body can't keep running hard forever. Like the seasons, there are times when you exert and grow, and times when you rest. You may not be at your declared destination yet, but that doesn't matter right now. You've S.C.O.R.E.D! Now it's time to **S**peculate on what worked, **C**elebrate your new self, **O**perate from a position of strength, **R**ejuvenate from your journey, and **E**valuate where to go from here.

Speculate on What Worked for You

You've made it to the finish line, and you're ready to sit down and enjoy your success. So let's speculate about what helped you get to this point in your journey while the memory is still new. What made you successful? What steps did you take that moved you past your comfort zone and led you to the success you are realizing today? Think about these past twelve weeks and about the person you have become.

What are the differences in your habits between then and now? Recognize where you've come, because that gives you security for who you are today. Acknowledge the struggle and the success—most of all, acknowledge the dream. You set out to accomplish a task, and through mental, physical, and spiritual force, you made it happen. How impressive is that?

Celebrate Your New Self

This is the moment you've been waiting for. Celebrate your efforts! Purchase your new outfit! Strut your stuff! It's time to reward yourself and do something that you've been looking forward to these past few months of hard work and discipline. Your reward was that motivation dangling in front of you when you wanted to give up. So take some time and relish this moment. Celebrate and relax. Give yourself a pat on the back—you deserve it.

Operate from a Position of Strength

This is a friendly reminder to keep your healthy habits going. Just because you reached your goal, that doesn't mean you can revert to your old routine. You can certainly splurge for a few days and take some time off from exercising, but I guarantee you, your tummy will ache after a few fat-laden, sugar-filled meals. Your body will crave movement, and your mind will miss the discipline. So continue operating; don't stop and don't think for one second that slacking off for an extended period is acceptable.

Remind yourself how hard you worked to lose 1 pound of fat, and remember how easy it is to gain that pound back—and then some. Most people who lose weight will gain their weight back because they overexercised and overdieted to exhaustion, then reverted to out-of-control habits. Avoid joining that statistic by continuing your healthy operations.

Rejuvenate, Rest, and Reward Yourself

Before you start creating new goals, rejuvenate. This does not mean you go on an eating binge for two weeks. It means you mindfully eat and move for the next couple weeks without pressure to attain a certain goal, with a specific deadline. You have to give yourself a break because if you don't, you will be driving on empty. So take this time to enjoy a few glasses of wine, an hour of extra sleep, and a spoonful of sugar in your coffee.

This is when the flexibility in your No More Excuses plan kicks in. You don't always have to be "on"—you just have to be on most of the time. Now you rejuvenate and refresh before you tackle new goals ahead.

Evaluate Your New Potential

This is where the fun begins again. Where do you want to go from here? Do you want to lose additional weight? Do you want to increase your running distance to a half-marathon? Do you want to get abdominal definition or compete in a fitness contest? What do you want to do? Think about your next physical goal, because if you don't continue to strive for something bigger, better, or longer, complacency will set in and you will slowly return to your old habits.

At this point you should be feeling empowered by the No More Excuses program and have mastered your S.P.E.E.D., your S.T.R.I.V.E., and now your S.C.O.R.E.

CONCLUSION

Your future is in your hands.

It's up to you to utilize the knowledge in this book and apply it in your daily life. No one is going to write down your goals, create your plan, and hang your action calendar. No one is going to cook your meals, organize your schedule, perform your workouts, or force you to do anything you don't want to do.

It's all up to you.

I've always believed in the power of choice and the immeasurable strength found in the faith to achieve intended goals. You must believe in your abilities before you become what you seek to accomplish. As I've repeated several times throughout this book, thoughts always turn into things. It's not easy to keep one's faith, after all, so many of us have become frustrated by the endless weight-loss cycle and are quietly convinced that we failed before we began!

I hope after reading this book you believe you can do it. You can be healthy without sacrificing your professional and personal life. You don't have to starve yourself or follow an unrealistic lifestyle. You don't have to give up your favorite foods or banish carbohydrates, abolish alcohol, or eliminate sugar from your life. All you have to do is be balanced but flexible. Challenge yourself by changing your habits slowly. Work in increments of three days, three weeks, and three months and give yourself time to transform. There is no greater gift than realizing your power to change your destiny simply by changing the way you see the world. You can either live passively behind your past failures and present excuses, or you can live aggressively by speeding, striving, and scoring toward a meaningful goal! It's not easy, but I promise you, it is worth it.

ACKNOWLEDGMENTS

This book could not have been written without the continuous support and encouragement of my husband, David Casler. Not only did he patiently help coparent our three young sons (ages 5, 4, and 2 at the time of this writing), but he always believed in me and my passion for health and fitness.

To my parents, Francis and Caroline Kang, who taught me about hard work, perseverance, love, compassion, and faith. Thank you for your positive example and unconditional belief in me. To my ever-supportive grandparents, George and Caridad Aducayen, and my family members, Eddie and Kristine Aducayen, Dominic Kang, Christine Enero, and Angeline Houston: You have all played an integral role in nourishing my passion and putting up with my birthday parties at the gym. Special thanks to my closest friends, Dave Slagle, Brian Woo, Borina Mak, Ana Sneed, and Araceli Wedderburn: If I ever need motivation, an understanding voice, or a good vent, all of you are on speed dial! To my Fitness Without Borders directors, especially our original team comprised of Stephanie

Quok, Dan Thompson, McCain Crow, Rodney Black, Hilary Herndon, Joseph Freschi, and Joe Ynostronza: Thank you for helping me build a nonprofit from passion and persistence. Thank you to all my artistic friends who helped put this book together, including clothing designer Elisabetta Rogiani, photographers James Patrick, Mike Byerly, and Jaymi Britten and illustrator Louis Dorman. Lastly, to my children, Christian, Nicholas, and Gabriel, as well as my step-children, Sydney, Piper, and Teddy: I thank God each day for giving me the gift of your presence in my life.

To my No Excuse Mom (NEM) family, including my long-time friend Lori Hare who cofounded the online group page. To our original NEM group page administrators: Shannon Link, Stephanie Stafford, Lorna Pope, Ashley Avila Aquino, Ay Carter, Gioia Aw, and Jaylene Lawrence. It's not easy managing thousands of women, but you do it freely and we are so thankful for your efforts. To our original hardworking regional managers: Jennifer Dillon, Barbie Caulder, Sherilyn Taylor, Nikeda Skanes, Katie Myers, Veronica Davila, Jessica Cordova, Jennifer Rowell, Juanita Verdin, Sarah Floyd, Leslee-Ann Martell, and Paulette Go. You are incredible leaders who are showing our next generation what passion and purpose look like. To our enthusiastic local leaders—there are definitely too many to list!—thank you for hosting free workouts and making a positive difference in your communities. To our helpful advisory board, our national fitness pros Vanessa Campos and Jules Rosenthal, and our nutritionists Diane Kazer and Felicia Newell, thank you for sharing your expertise, knowledge, and most of all your incredible, never-ending energy. Thousands of women are benefiting throughout the world because of the personal efforts of our NEM family. We are showing the world that health starts at home and comes in various shapes, sizes, and ages.

To my incredible team, including book agent Brandi Bowles, editor Leah Miller, marketing manager Christina Foxley, publicist

Lauren Cook, and my manager, Antranig Balian: Thank you for all the guidance and encouragement you've given this first-time author! I've always envisioned publishing a book, but I never imagined partnering with Crown, Foundry, and Mortar Media in writing a program I am truly proud of.

APPENDIX

POSTURE QUIZ AND STRETCHES FOR BETTER POSTURE

It is rare to find someone who has perfect posture. But bad posture is a hard habit to break; you need to be conscious of all your actions, especially involuntary ones that are enforced by surrounding muscles. Yet poor posture can lead to lower back pain, among other problems. When you suffer from lower back pain, as nearly 80 percent of the U.S. population does, it can prevent you from living a fulfilling and active life.

Excess weight, poor posture, and muscle imbalances all increase your chances of bodily injury. According to Dr. James Rainville, a renowned expert in back pain and chief of physical medicine and rehabilitation at New England Baptist Hospital in Boston, the best way to prevent and protect yourself from back pain is strength training, stretching, and aerobic exercise. Dr. Rainville believes that exercise can often help retrain the nervous system to desensitize overactive nerves.

Additionally, if you have bad posture, you cannot develop your core strength. And, as was discussed in Chapter 6, a strong core translates into a strong body. Further, a strong body is not an imbalanced body. So fix your posture and focus on strengthening those weak muscles.

POSTURE QUIZ

If you have bad posture, you need to nip it in the bud. If you don't know if you do, here is a quick quiz:

1. Does your occupation require you to sit most of the day?
   A. Yes
   B. No

2. Do you carry most of your body weight in your upper body?
   A. Yes
   B. No

3. Do your shoulders slope forward?
  A. Yes
  B. No

4. Does your belly protrude out?
  A. Yes
  B. No

5. Do you have any lower back pain?
  A. Yes
  B. No

6. Do your hamstrings get tight?
  A. Yes
  B. No

> If you answered mostly As, you have a postural deviation. Don't be discouraged; many people suffer from imbalanced muscles, stemming from excess sitting, playing video games, and being generally inactive. Your posture can be fixed by stretching and strengthening the tight muscles.

Stretches for Better Posture

Fixing your posture also assists in generating confidence and making you appear slimmer. When you stand tall with your shoulders back and your hips squared, you look longer, stronger, and more assertive. Many women complain of having a flabby belly, but as soon as they stand straight and engage their tummy, they look 5 pounds lighter. So, let's begin: Chest up! Shoulders back! Tummy in! Hips squared!

1. **Start stretching out your tight muscles and strengthening your weak muscles. Be more cognizant of your posture by**

keeping your chest up, shoulders back, chin up, hips squared, and feet forward.

2. Combating your muscle imbalances will require you to perform a variety of stretch and strength exercises. These exercises will repair your posture by extending tight muscles and toughening weak muscles. If performed several times a week you can build a stronger core, strengthen your lumbar region, and decrease your chances of injury. See which of the following sounds most like you and take corrective action:

UPPER CROSSED SYNDROME

People who struggle with an upper crossed syndrome usually have weak chest and back muscles and tight shoulders. If you have a desk job, drive often, or have a larger chest area, you may be slouching forward more often than you realize and creating muscle imbalances. If you look at the diagram, you can see the body's alignment is off-kilter; now imagine applying weight onto a body that is imbalanced. Like a rotting tree trunk or a house with a poor foundation,

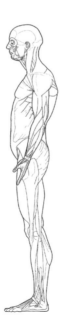

it will "break"—it's not a matter of if but *when*. You need to stretch out the tight muscles and strengthen the weak muscles. If you have an upper crossed syndrome, your stretching should focus on opening up your chest. Your strength training should focus on building your chest and back muscles.

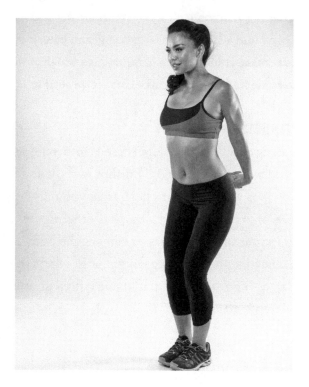

CHEST STRETCH

Clasp your hands behind your back and slowly lift your arms away from your back and up toward the ceiling. Hold this stretch for 10 to 30 seconds.

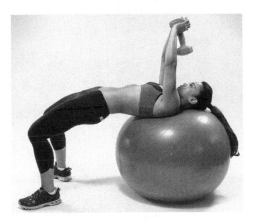

LYING DB PULLOVER

Position your upper back on a firm stability ball or bench, and squeeze your glutes.

Place a dumbbell between both hands and slowly lower the weight above and over your head. Perform three sets of 12 to 15 repetitions.

....

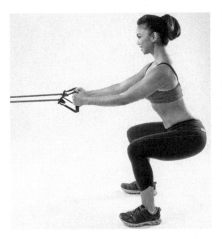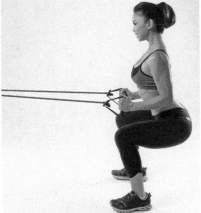

SQUATTING RB BACK ROW

Loop a resistance band around an object at your chest or shoulder height. Stand facing the band in a squatted position. Grab the handles with each hand and reach forward with your arms shoulder-distance apart. Pull the band until your elbows pass the line of your back. Slowly release.

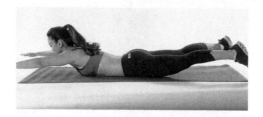

SUPERMAN

Lie facedown on a mat. Extend your arms out in front of you and raise your upper and lower halves. Squeeze your glutes and tighten your lower back. Hold for 30 to 60 seconds and repeat three times.

LOWER CROSSED SYNDROME

Lower crossed syndrome is a muscle imbalance that causes tightness in the lower back as well as weakness in the glutes, the lower back, and abdominal muscles. If you notice your body mimics the image below, it's important to begin stretching your tight muscles and strengthening your weak muscles.

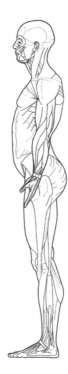

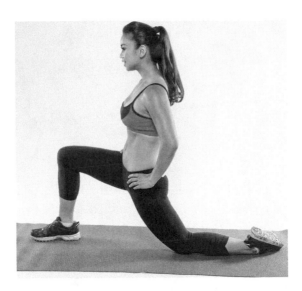

HIP FLEXOR

Kneel in a lunge position and open up your back hip. Hold for 25 to 30 seconds and change sides.

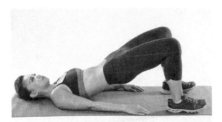 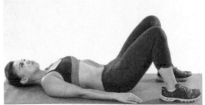

GLUTE BRIDGE

Lie faceup on a mat with your knees bent. Lift your hips off the ground while squeezing your hamstrings, glutes, and lower back. Hold for 30 to 60 seconds.

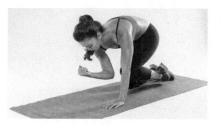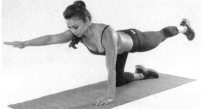

BIRD DOG

Get down on all fours on a mat, keeping your hips squared, core tight, and spine neutral. At the same time, draw your right arm and left leg in; then lift and extend both. Hold for 30 to 60 seconds, then switch sides.

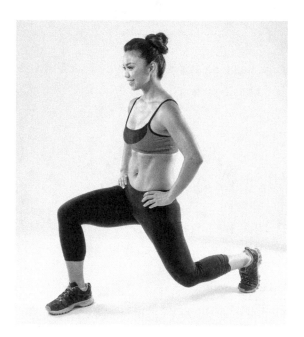

FRONT LUNGE

Stand up straight, with your feet shoulder-width apart, chest up, shoulders back, and core tight. Step forward with your left foot and lower your right knee toward the floor. Push off your left foot to return to the starting position. Repeat with the other leg.

PLANK

This is hands down my favorite exercise for the abdominal region. It works on your deepest core muscle, your transverse abdominals (TVA), as well as your lower back. Begin in a hands and knees position on a mat with your hands directly under your shoulders, fingers facing forward. Now, choose one of three different plank levels: The first is on your hands with your knees on the mat; the second is on your hands with your knees off the mat; and the third (the most traditional stance) is on your elbows with your knees off the mat. Keep a neutral spine and hips squared. Use a timer and measure how long you can hold the plank position. Every week increase your time by 15 seconds. I perform this exercise in the beginning, middle, or end of my abdominal workouts. It doesn't matter when you perform the plank; just make sure you incorporate it daily into your exercise regimen.

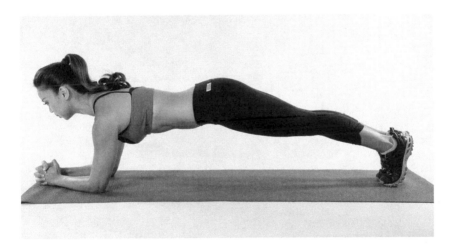

STRENGTH-TRAINING EXERCISES FOR CHAPTER 6

Please note that each exercise can be altered by the use of equipment. You can also increase difficulty by alternating arms or standing on one leg.

PLYOMETRICS

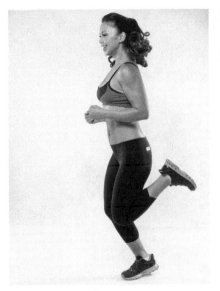

BUTT KICK
Run in place, bringing your heels to your glutes.

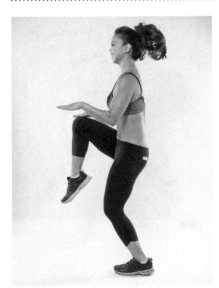
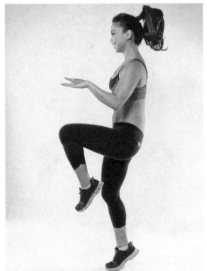

HIGH KNEE
Run in place, bringing your knees up to your chest as high as you can.

MOUNTAIN CLIMBER

Begin in a push-up position on a mat (see page 251). Bring your right knee to your chest, keeping your left foot on the mat. Switch feet in midair.

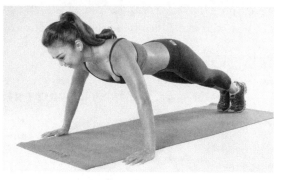

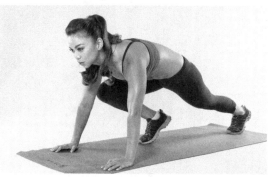

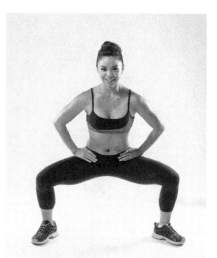

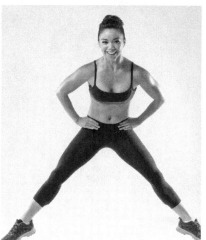

BW SQUAT JUMP

Begin in a squat position, jump up, and land in a squat position.

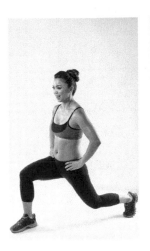
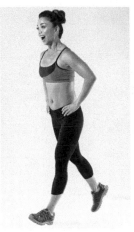
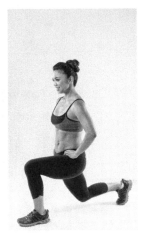

BW LUNGE JUMP

Begin in a lunge position (see page 244), then jump up and swap leg positions in midair, while keeping your torso straight.

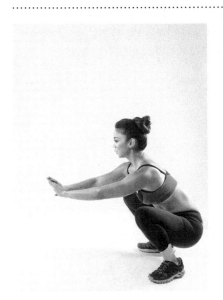
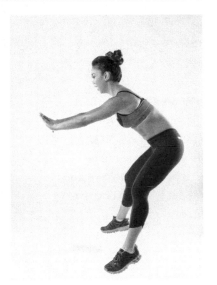

FROG JUMP

Begin in a deep squat position with your knees bent and buttocks lowered toward the ground. Jump forward and land in the same deep squat position.

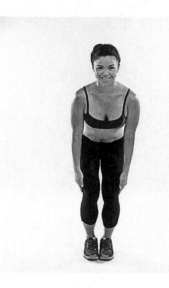
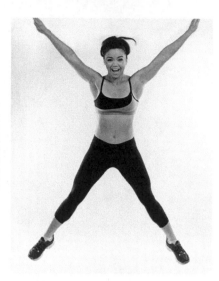

BW STAR JUMP

Begin in a relaxed stance with your feet together and hold your arms close to the body. Squat down halfway and explode back up as high as possible with your arms and legs fully extended. Descend back into starting position.

BW STEP-UP

Place your right foot on a stable chair. Stand straight up with your leg fully extended. Step down and repeat with the opposite foot.

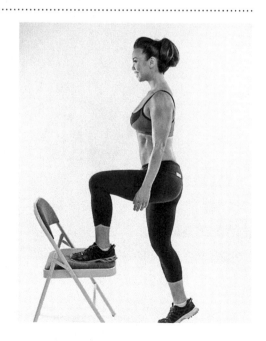

CHEST

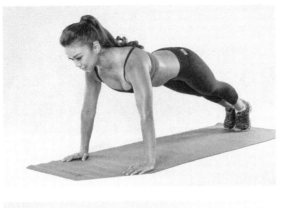

BW PUSH-UP

Begin in a hands and knees position on a mat with your hands directly under your shoulders, fingers facing forward. If you can, raise your knees off the floor. Slowly bend your elbows, lowering your body toward the mat, and push up with your chest while keeping your core engaged.

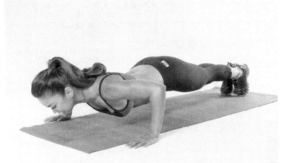

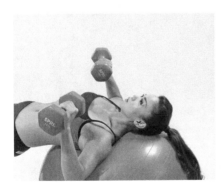 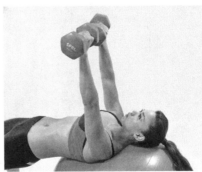

LYING DB CHEST PRESS

Lie down with your upper back on a stability ball and your feet on the floor. Hold a dumbbell in each hand by your chest with your palms facing forward. Press the dumbbells up until your elbows are straight. Slowly lower the dumbbells by bending your elbows until they reach a bit past 90 degrees.

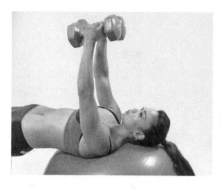
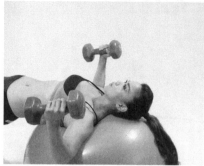

LYING DB CHEST FLY

Lie down with your upper back on a stability ball and your feet on the floor. Hold a dumbbell in each hand with your arms straight, directly above your chest, and your palms facing each other. Slowly lower your arms until they become level with your chest, then squeeze your chest to raise the dumbbells back up to the starting position.

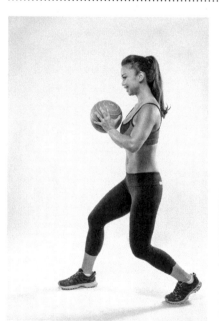
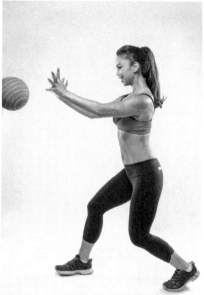

MB CHEST PASS

Stand 3 to 4 feet away from a partner or wall. Bring a medicine ball to your chest, then throw the ball as hard as possible to your partner or at the wall.

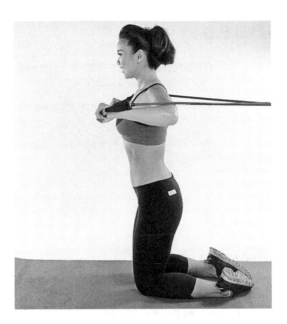

RB CHEST PRESS

Loop the center of a resistance band around a stable object at your chest or shoulder height. Stand or kneel facing away from the band and grab the handles with each hand. Position your arms at 90 degree angles with your palms facing down. Extend your arms outward, pushing through your chest without locking your elbows. In a controlled motion, return your arms back to the starting position and repeat.

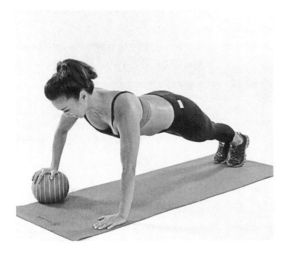

MB PUSH-UP

Get into a push-up position, resting your right hand on a medicine ball. Lower your body toward the ground, bending your arms nearly 90 degrees, then raise yourself back up to the starting position. Switch arms and repeat.

SHOULDERS

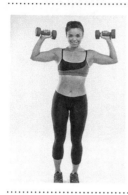

DB SHOULDER PRESS

Hold dumbbells on each side of your head with your elbows below your wrists. Press upward until your arms are extended, then slowly bring back the dumbbells to the starting position.

DB SQUATTED ALTERNATING SHOULDER PRESS

In a squatted position, hold a dumbbell in each hand with your arms at 90 degree angles beside your head. Your palms should be facing forward and your elbows pointed out. Extend one arm to press the dumbbell straight up, keeping your other arm in place. Then slowly bring back the dumbbell to the starting position and repeat with the opposite side.

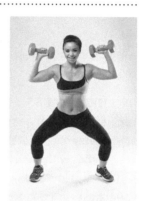

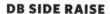

DB ONE-LEGGED SHOULDER PRESS

Engage your core and balance on one foot. Hold dumbbells on each side of your head with your elbows below your wrist. Press upward until your arms are extended, then slowly bring back the dumbbells to the starting position.

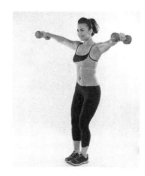

DB SIDE RAISE

Stand with your feet shoulder-width apart and hold dumbbells down by your sides. Slowly raise both dumbbells up to about eye level. Lower and repeat.

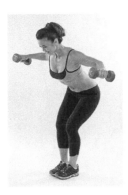

DB REVERSE FLY

Holding two dumbbells, bend over with your arms hanging down in front of you. Keep your knees slightly bent and your back straight. Raise your arms until they are level with your shoulders and pause. Lower arms back to the starting position and repeat.

DB STANDING UPRIGHT ROW

Stand with your feet slightly apart and hold dumbbells with an overhand grip. Your hands should be shoulder-width apart. Draw the dumbbells up toward your collarbone by bending your elbows. Your wrists flex as the weights rise.

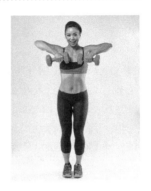

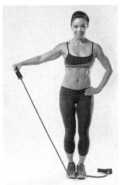

RB STANDING ONE-ARM LATERAL RAISE

Stand on a resistance band so that tension begins at arm's length. Grasp one handle with one hand and raise your arm to the side until your elbow is shoulder height. Repeat with your other arm.

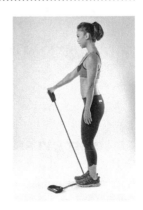

RB STANDING ONE-ARM FRONT RAISE

Stand on a resistance band so that tension begins at arm's length. Grasp the handle with one hand and raise your arm to the front until your elbow is shoulder height. Repeat with your other arm.

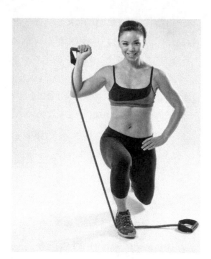

RB ONE-ARM SHOULDER PRESS WITH LUNGE
Stand in a lunge position with your right foot on a resistance band and your right hand holding one handle of the band level with your ears. Perform a lunge (see page 244) and press the band up above your head as you rise to the starting position. Switch sides.

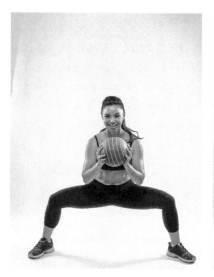 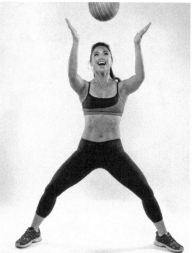

MB SQUAT OVERHEAD THROW
Begin in a squat position with a medicine ball at your chest/neck level. As you come out of the squat and rise, throw the ball overhead and then catch it in a squat position.

ARMS

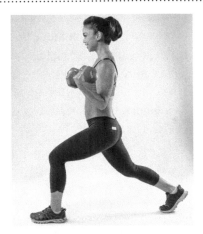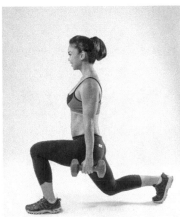

DB BICEP CURL WITH LUNGE

Stand with your feet shoulder-width apart and your hands holding dumbbells at your sides. Simultaneously lunge (see page 244) and curl the dumbbells in front of your chest with your palms up. Slowly reverse to return to the starting position. Repeat with the other leg.

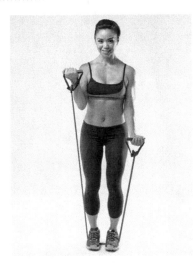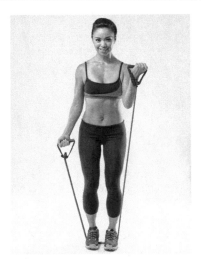

RB STANDING ALTERNATING BICEP CURL

Place a resistance band securely under your feet and stand erect with your feet slightly apart. Hold one handle in each hand, palms facing up. Curl one arm up toward your shoulder at a time, keeping your elbows close to your sides. Slowly lower your arm to the start position, then repeat with the opposite arm.

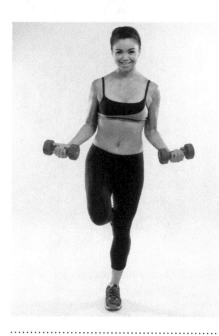

DB ONE-LEGGED STANDING BICEP CURL

Standing on one leg, engage your core and hold the dumbbells with your palms facing forward. In a controlled motion, raise the dumbbells toward your shoulders, flexing at the top, then extend and repeat.

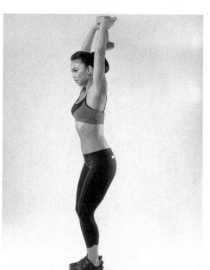 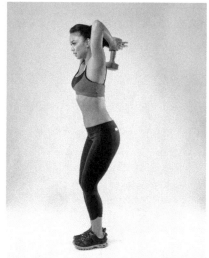

DB STANDING TRICEP EXTENSION

Standing with your feet together and a slight bend in your knees, position one dumbbell over your head with both hands under the inner plate (heart-shaped grip). With your elbows over your head, lower your forearms behind your upper arms by flexing your elbows. Raise the dumbbell over your head while keeping your elbows steady and close to your ears.

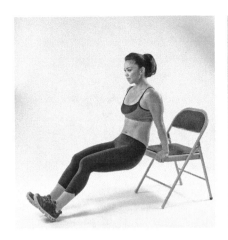
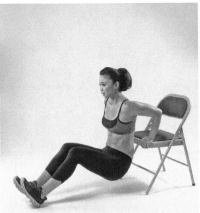

BW CHAIR TRICEPS DIP

Place your palms on the edge of a chair and extend your feet forward. Lower your body by bending your arms until a slight stretch is felt in your chest or shoulders, or your rear end touches the floor. Raise your body by extending your arms without locking your elbows.

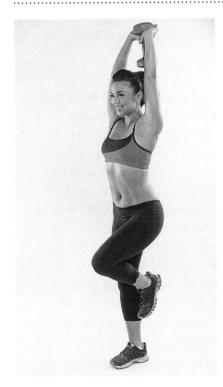

DB ONE-LEGGED OVERHEAD TRICEP EXTENSION

Engage your core and hold a dumbbell over your head with two hands. Balance yourself and slowly raise one foot off the ground. Bend/lower your arms approximately 90 degrees, then extend straight up and repeat.

BACK

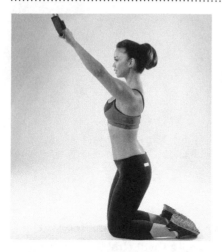 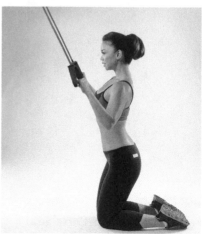

KNEELING RB LAT PULL-DOWN

Loop a resistance band over a high stationary object. Kneel facing the resistance band. With your arms extended overhead, hands wider than shoulder-width apart, grab the handles with both hands. Pull your hands down, squeezing your shoulder blades together, until your hands are around chest height. Slowly release.

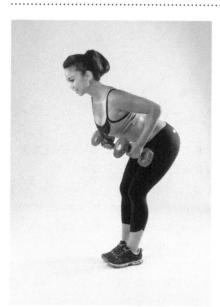

STANDING DB BENT-OVER BACK ROW

With a dumbbell on either side of you, stand with your feet slightly apart. Grab the dumbbells with your palms facing inward. With your knees slightly bent, bend at your waist and let the dumbbells hang down in front of you. In a slow, controlled movement, pull the dumbbells up to your lower abdomen and squeeze your back at the top. Slowly lower the dumbbells until your arms are fully extended.

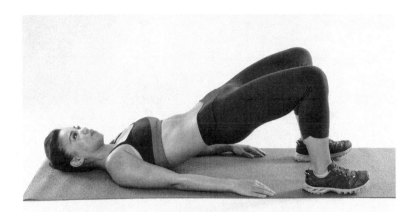

LYING BACK HIP EXTENSION

Lie on your back with your feet on the floor, your knees bent, and your arms by your side, palms down. Raise your hips up, squeezing your glutes and engaging your core. Hold for several seconds, then return to the starting position.

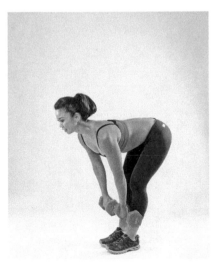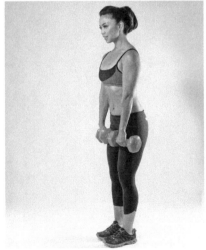

DB DEAD LIFT

With a dumbbell in each hand, stand with your feet slightly apart. With your knees slightly bent, lower the dumbbells to the top or sides of your feet by bending at your waist. Lift the dumbbells by extending your hips and waist until you're standing upright.

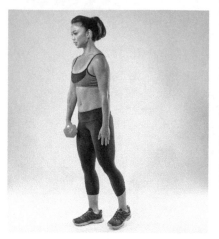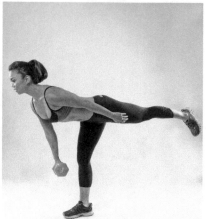

DB ONE-LEGGED DEAD LIFT

Grab one dumbbell and hold it in front of you. Standing on one leg, raise the other leg behind you, toes facing down, as you lower the dumbbell toward your standing foot. Lift the dumbbell by extending your hips and waist until you're standing upright with both legs on the ground. Switch sides.

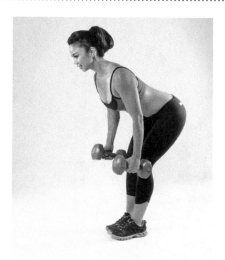

DB BENT-OVER ROW

Stand with your feet slightly apart. Bend over while keeping your back straight. Pull the dumbbells up toward the sides of your body by bending your arms.

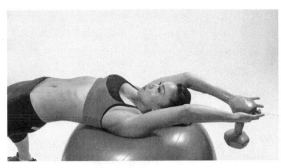

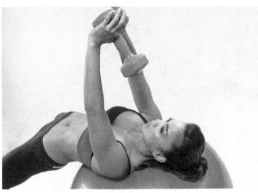

LYING DB BACK PULLOVER

Lie on your upper back on a stability ball, keeping your feet on the floor and flexing your hips slightly. With both hands, grasp one dumbbell under the inner plate. Position the dumbbell over your chest with your elbows slightly bent. Lower the dumbell above your head while keeping your elbows stable. Pull the dumbbell up and over your chest.

CORE

BW V-UP

From a plank position on a mat, raise your hips up toward the ceiling, hold, then return to a plank position.

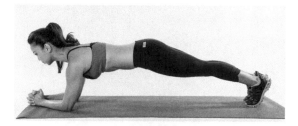

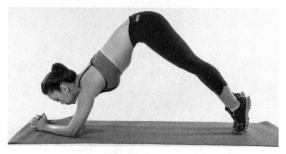

BW SIDE PLANK

Lie on your side on a mat, with your upper leg directly on top of your lower leg. Place your forearm on the mat under your shoulder, perpendicular to your body. Raise your hips off the mat, hold, then lower to the starting position. Switch sides.

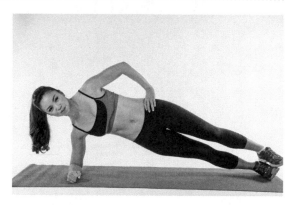

SUPERMAN

Lie facedown with your arms and legs extended. Squeeze your glutes and tighten your lower back.

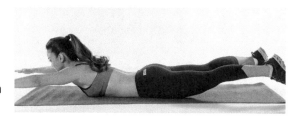

TOE TOUCH

Lie on your back on a mat with your legs in the air at about a 90 degree angle. With your arms extended, raise your upper back off the mat and crunch up toward your toes.

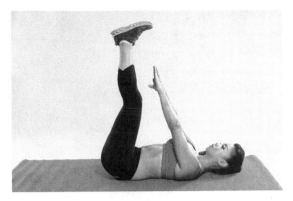

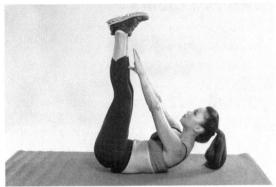

BW BICYCLE CRUNCH

Lie faceup on a mat and position your hands behind your neck. Pretend you are holding an orange under your chin. Bring one knee toward your chest while reaching your opposite elbow toward it. Alternate sides.

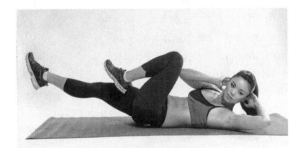

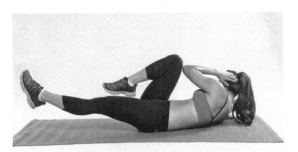

BW RUSSIAN TWIST

(Note: This exercise can be performed using no weights or with a dumbbell or medicine ball.) Sit with your heels on a mat and your back slightly lowered. Without rounding out your spine, turn side to side, touching the ground on each side of your hip.

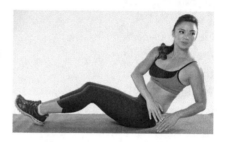

BW REVERSE CRUNCH

Lie faceup on a mat with your knees bent, feet flat on the floor, and your hands at your sides. Lift your legs straight up toward the ceiling and decline slowly without touching the ground.

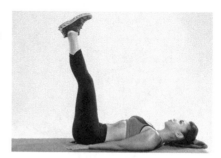

BW FLUTTER KICK

Lying flat on your back, place your arms by your sides or beneath you for support. Extend your legs out and raise your feet several inches off the ground. Engage your core, then begin making small, rapid, scissorlike motions with your legs.

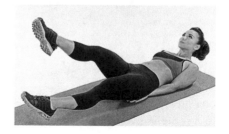

MB CURL-UP

Lying flat on your back with your legs slightly bent and your heels to the ground, hold a medicine ball over your head. Slowly curl up into a seated position while raising the ball above your head, then decline to the starting position and repeat.

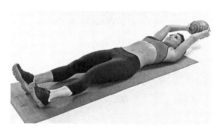

LEGS

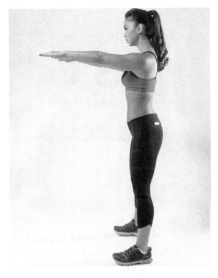

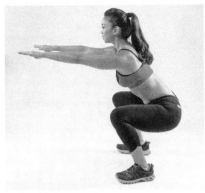

BW SQUAT

Stand with your feet facing forward and shoulder-width apart. Bend your hips back and allow your knees to bend forward slightly, keeping your back straight. Descend until your thighs are just past parallel to the floor. Reverse and extend your hips and knees until your legs are straight.

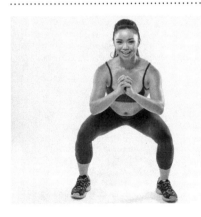

BW SQUAT KICK

Stand with your feet facing forward and shoulder-width apart. Squat down by bending your hips back while allowing your knees to bend forward slightly. While returning to the standing position, kick one leg and then squat as your leg returns to the floor. Switch legs.

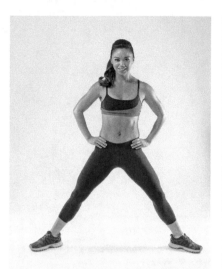 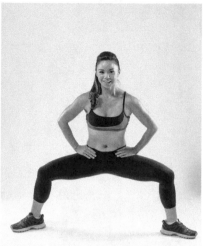

BW PLIE SQUAT

Stand with your legs 2 to 3 feet apart, toes turned out; place your hands on your hips. Push your hips back and lower your body until your thighs are parallel to the floor. Slowly ascend to the starting position.

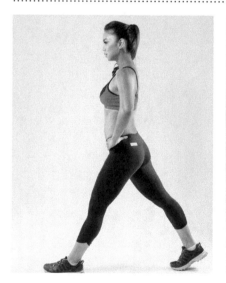 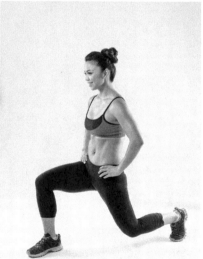

BW LUNGE

Position your feet shoulder-width apart and extend one leg forward. Bend your front leg to a 90 degree angle. Push through your heels and straighten your leg back to the starting position.

CURTSY LUNGE

Stand with your feet shoulder-width apart. Lunge diagonally backward with your right foot crossing the back of your left leg, bending both knees at 90 degrees. Straighten your legs and return to the starting position.

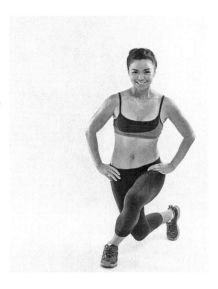

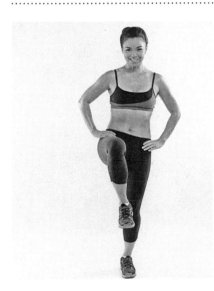

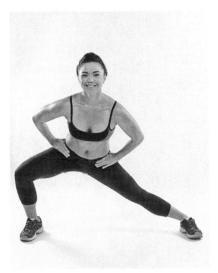

BW SIDE LUNGE

Stand with your feet shoulder-width apart. Extend your right knee up toward your chest, then land in a right lunge toward the floor. Make sure your right knee does not go past your toes and your left leg is nearly straight. Raise your right leg back into the starting position and switch legs.

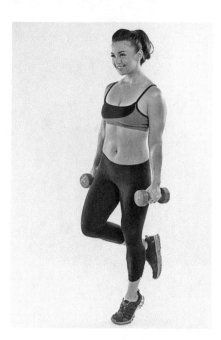

DB CALF RAISE

Stand with your feet shoulder-width apart and hold a dumbbell in each hand. Raise your heels off the ground until you feel your calves contract. You can do this either with both feet on the ground or alternating on one leg.

STRETCHING EXERCISES FOR CHAPTER 6

NECK

Place your right hand on the top of your head and slowly tilt it to the right until you feel a gentle pressure. Repeat on the opposite side.

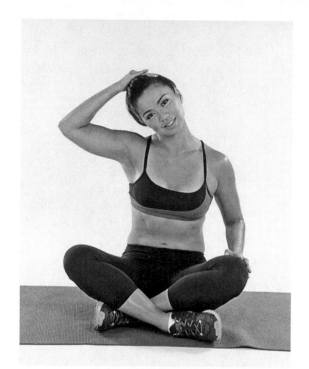

BACK

Lie faceup on a mat, stretching your arms out to the side at shoulder height, palms up. While keeping your shoulders on the mat, bring your right knee up and lower it to the opposite side of the body. Hold it down with your left hand and then switch sides.

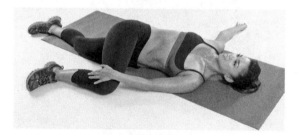

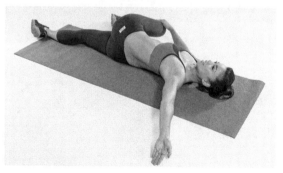

LOWER BACK

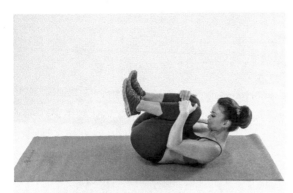

Lie on your back on a mat and bring both knees to your chest. Pull your knees down toward your chest and lift your head forward, chin toward your chest. Hold.

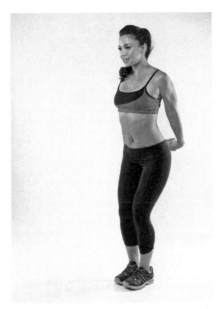

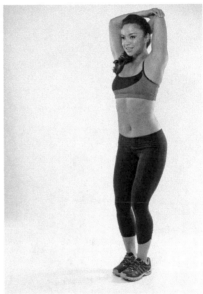

CHEST

Stand tall or sit upright. Interlace your fingers behind your back and straighten your arms.

TRICEPS

Raise one arm overhead. Position your forearm as close as possible to your upper arm. Grasp your elbow overhead with your other hand. Pull your elbow back toward your head. Repeat with your other arm.

SHOULDERS

Position one arm across your body.
Place your opposite hand above
your elbow and press against your
chest. Repeat with your other arm.

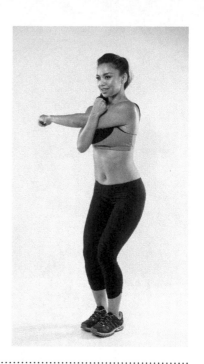

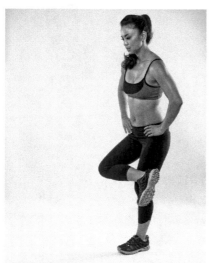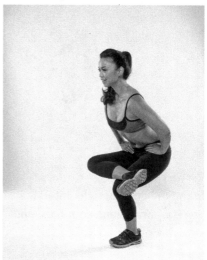

STANDING GLUTES

Stand and touch a wall or a stationary object for balance, if necessary.
Place the outside of your foot across your stationary upper leg and sit into
the stretch. Repeat with your other leg.

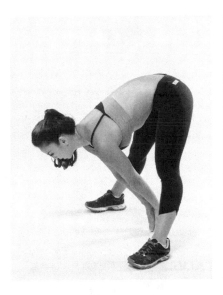

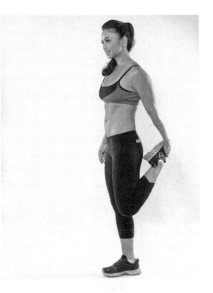

HAMSTRINGS

Stand with your feet wider than your shoulders with your toes pointed diagonally outward. Slowly bend forward from the waist, bringing your hands toward your right foot and keeping your back flat. Repeat on the other side.

STANDING QUADS

Stand and touch a wall or a stationary object for balance. Grasp the top ankle or forefoot of one leg behind you. Pull your ankle or forefoot to your rear end. Repeat with your other leg.

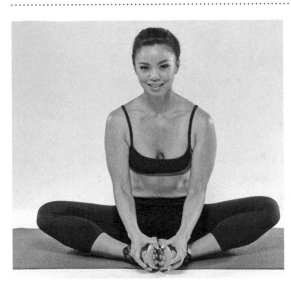

INNER THIGHS

Sit up tall on a mat with the soles of your feet pressed together. Place your hands on your ankles, and drop your knees as comfortably as they will go. Pull your abdominals in and lean forward with your hips.

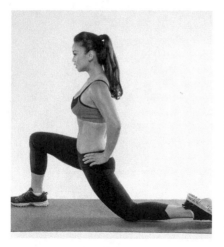

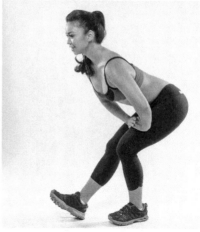

HIP FLEXOR

Lunge forward with your knee on a mat. Place your hands on your hips and push your hips forward. Repeat with your other leg.

CALVES

Stand with one leg slightly in front of the other and bent at the knee. Bend forward at the hips and put your weight on your bent leg. Repeat with your other leg.

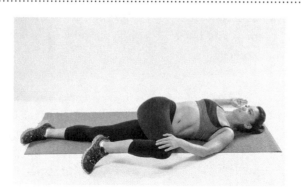

LYING SPINAL TWIST

Lie on your back with your arms horizontally stretched out in line with your shoulders. Bend your right knee and bring your foot close to your hip. Swing your knee to the left until the left knee touches the ground. Simultaneously, turn your head to the right and look at your right palm.

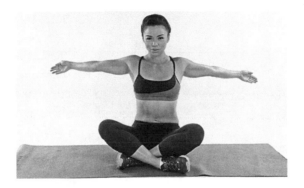

SEATED ARM CIRCLES

Stand or sit and stretch your arms out to your sides so that your body is in a T formation. Hold your arms stiff and push your muscles out tight as if you were pushing against something. Let your palms face out, with your thumbs pointing upward. Make small circle motions backward with your arms. Then face your palms in, point your thumbs down, and reverse to forward arm circles. Do about 15 to 20 arm circles in each direction.

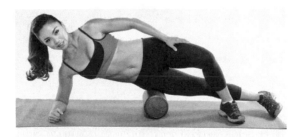

FOAM ROLLER IT BAND

Lie on your side on a mat, support your body weight with your legs and arms as shown, and place a foam roller under the upper, outside portion of your bottom thigh. Apply weight and allow the foam roller to run up and down the side of your thigh. Repeat on the opposite side.

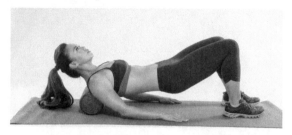

SMR UPPER BACK

Lie faceup on a mat. Position a foam roller under your upper back and rear shoulders. Keep your head up and feet on the mat. Apply weight and allow the foam roller to roll up toward your neck and down toward your mid-back.

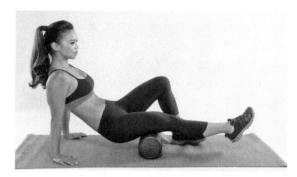

SMR HAMSTRINGS

Lie faceup on a mat. Position a foam roller underneath your thigh, while supporting your body weight with your legs and arms as shown. Apply weight and allow the foam roller to roll up toward your glutes and down toward your knees. Repeat on the other leg.

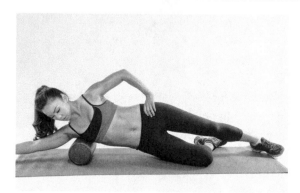

LATISSIMUS DORSI

Lie on your side on a mat, support your body with your legs and arms as shown, and lie with a foam roller on the wings of your body. Apply weight and allow the foam roller to run down toward your waist and up toward your armpit. Repeat on the other side.

YOGA POSES

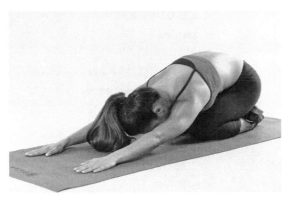

CHILD'S POSE

Kneel on a mat. Touch your big toes together and sit on your heels, then separate your knees about as wide as your hips. Extend your arms in front of your body and sit your hips back toward your heels. Reach your forehead toward the floor.

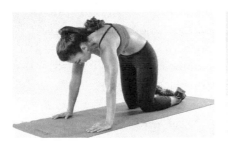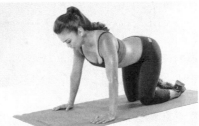

CAT-COW STRETCH

Get on all fours on a mat. Breathing deeply, arch your back like a cat. Gently return to resting position. Now, allow your torso to bend toward the floor, forming a downward curve.

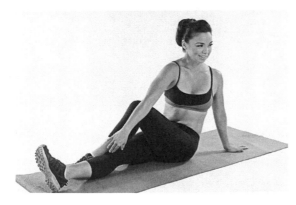

SEATED SPINAL TWIST

In a seated position, place your right knee on the outside of your left leg. Twist your torso to the left, placing your right arm outside your right knee.

GROCERY LIST

PROTEIN
beef (lean cuts)
buffalo
chicken breast
cod fillets
cottage cheese (low-fat)
crab
egg whites or substitutes
ground turkey
haddock
lobster
orange roughy
salmon
shrimp
tilapia
trout
tuna
turkey bacon
turkey breast
wild game meat

SOURCES OF PROTEIN FOR VEGANS
beans
chickpeas
edamame
leafy greens
lentils
nuts
peas
quinoa
seeds (sesame, sunflower, poppy)
soy milk
tempeh
tofu

CARBOHYDRATES
Complex
barley
beans (black, kidney)
bread (whole-wheat)
brown rice
buckwheat
bulgur
cereal (high-fiber)
corn
couscous
lentils
millet
oatmeal
pasta (whole-wheat)
popcorn
potatoes
pumpkin
squash
tortillas (whole-wheat)

Vegetables
artichokes
arugula
asparagus
avocados
bell peppers
broccoli
Brussels sprouts
cabbage
cauliflower
celery
corn
eggplant
grape tomatoes
green beans

jicama
kale
leeks
lemons
limes
mushrooms
olives
onions
pumpkin
romaine lettuce
salad greens
shallots
snow peas
spinach
squash
tomatoes (regular and Roma)
turnips
water chestnuts
zucchini

Simple
apples
bananas
bread (white)
carrots
figs
fruit juice
grapefruit
guava
high-fructose corn syrup
honey
kiwi
mangoes
maple syrup

milk
molasses
nectarines
oranges
pasta (white)
pears
rhubarb
rice (white)
sugar
yogurt

DAIRY PRODUCTS
butter
cream and/or milk
feta cheese
goat cheese (mild)
Greek yogurt (plain or vanilla)
havarti cheese
Parmesan cheese
sour cream (low- or non-fat)

FATS
avocado
coconut
cold-water fish (salmon, mackerel, trout, tuna)
nuts (almonds, hazelnuts, pecans, walnuts)
oil (coconut, grapeseed, hemp, olive)
olives
peanuts
seeds (chia, pumpkin, sesame, sunflower)

INDEX